CHILD AND ADULT DEVELOPMENT

A PSYCHOANALYTIC INTRODUCTION FOR CLINICIANS

CRITICAL ISSUES IN PSYCHIATRY
An Educational Series for Residents and Clinicians

Series Editor: Sherwyn M. Woods, M.D., Ph.D.
University of Southern California School of Medicine
Los Angeles, California

A Continuation Order Plan is available for this series. A continuation order will bring
delivery of each new volume immediately upon publication. Volumes are billed only upon
actual shipment. For further information please contact the publisher.

CHILD AND ADULT DEVELOPMENT

A PSYCHOANALYTIC INTRODUCTION FOR CLINICIANS

CALVIN A. COLARUSSO, M.D.

University of California at San Diego
School of Medicine
La Jolla, California

PLENUM PRESS • NEW YORK AND LONDON

Library of Congress Cataloging-in-Publication Data

Colarusso, Calvin A.
    Child and adult development : a psychoanalytic introduction for
clinicians / Calvin A. Colarusso.
        p.   cm. -- (Critical issues in psychiatry)
    Includes bibliographical references and index.
    ISBN 0-306-44285-X
    1. Developmental psychology. 2. Psychoanalysis. 3. Life cycle,
Human. 4. Child psychology.   I. Title. II. Series.
    [DNLM: 1. Child Development. 2. Human Development.
3. Psychoanalysis.   BF 713 C683c]
RC506.C58   1992
155--dc20
DNLM/DLC
for Library of Congress   92-49740
                                                                   CIP

ISBN 0-306-44285-X

© 1992 Plenum Press, New York
A Division of Plenum Publishing Corporation
233 Spring Street, New York, N.Y. 10013

Teaching is a privilege.
This book is dedicated to those mental health
students and professionals who have allowed me
to touch their lives, in the process
greatly enriching my own.

Foreword

Developmental theory is the essence of any psychodynamic psychotherapy, and certainly of psychoanalysis. It is through an understanding of progressive life events, and the way these events relate to associated biological and social events, that we come to understand both psychopathology and psychological strengths.

For a long time we have needed a clinically oriented book that surveys normal development in both childhood and adulthood. This book should be particularly helpful to all mental health professionals whose daily work requires a constant awareness and appraisal of developmental issues. Dr. Colarusso has integrated and summarized a tremendous amount of theoretical, empirical, and clinical material in a format that makes it come alive through clinical examples.

This book should be of great interest to all students of human behavior as well as to seasoned clinicians.

SHERWYN M. WOODS, M.D., PH.D.

Preface

Each year as I gave a lecture series on child and adult development to the adult and child psychiatric residents at the University of California at San Diego, someone inevitably would ask, "Is there a book that I could understand that has all of this information in it?" I would reply that I did not know of any single source, but I could refer the person to many articles and books on development. The look of dissatisfaction on the resident's face was inevitably followed by, "Well, why don't you write one that will introduce us to development and help us with our patients?" I was slow to catch on but eventually got the message and decided to try.

I have closely followed the directions that were given me by my students. This book is intended to be an *introduction* to developmental theory. My intent was to present concepts of adult and child development in a way that would stimulate the reader to want to know more, to go beyond this book to others that treat various aspects of the field in more detail. In nearly every chapter I have suggested such books.

My second intent, again following the directions of my students, was to produce a book that would be *clinically relevant*. Therefore, the developmental concepts presented had to relate to the student's work with patients, to their assessment and treatment.

I hope that *Child and Adult Development* will have an audience beyond mental health students. More experienced clinicians who are not familiar with recent advances in developmental thinking may find this effort a convenient place to begin their update. Finally, those adults, professional or not, who are interested in enhancing their interactions with children and in understanding their own experience as human beings will find much of interest in these pages.

For me, developmental theory is perpetually exciting and of unending fascination because it comes closer to answering the questions "Who am I?" and "How do I find happiness?" than any other source I know.

CALVIN A. COLARUSSO, M.D.

Acknowledgments

Over the past 20 years or so, I have had the privilege of teaching developmental theory and its clinical application to more than 1,000 medical students, psychiatric residents, and other mental health students and professionals at the University of California at San Diego. Their interest in development stimulated me to write this book, and I would like to thank them for their inspiration. In particular, I would like to thank their current representatives, those child psychiatric residents and graduate students in psychology who were kind enough to read the manuscript and offer suggestions: Eve Dryfus, Steve Elig, Sandra Lee, Gina Livesay, Jim Manning, Carola Suarez-Orozco, Robert Solomon, and Peter Vic.

The manuscript was typed and edited by two young psychologists who are very close to my heart, Mary Ann and Rob Stieber, my daughter and son-in-law.

Very special thanks are reserved for Robert Nemiroff, friend, officemate, and coauthor for two decades. His concepts and creativity are evident throughout this book.

I would also like to thank Lewis Judd, Professor and Chairman of Psychiatry at the University of California at San Diego. Unfailingly supportive of my clinical and research efforts, he has provided an atmosphere in which critical thinking and new ideas flourish.

This is the third time I have had the privilege of working with Sherwyn M. Woods. Outstanding psychiatrist, analyst, educator, and editor, he suggested that Robert Nemiroff and I write *Adult Development* (1981), and reacted positively to our suggestion to publish *The Race against Time* (1985). When I began to conceptualize this book, I naturally thought of Sherwyn and Plenum Press.

This is the first time I have had the pleasure of working with Mariclaire Cloutier, Plenum's Medical and Social Sciences Editor. Her friendliness, intelligence, and flexibility have made a potentially difficult process very easy.

Finally, I would like to thank my loving wife, Jean, for her unambivalent encouragement of my efforts. She has given me the time and the freedom to pursue my work at my own pace. I hope I have returned the favor half as well.

Contents

The Stages of Development

Oral phase	0–18 months
Anal phase	1–3 years of age
Oedipal phase	3–6 years of age
Latency phase	6–12 years of age
Adolescent phase	12–20 years of age
Young adulthood	Ages 20–40
Middle adulthood	Ages 40–60
Late adulthood	Ages 60–80
Late late adulthood	Ages 80–

Note: The childhood phases were first described by Sigmund Freud; the adult stages by Erik Erikson.

CHAPTER 1

A Historical Overview and General Principles of Child Development

The purpose of this brief overview is to introduce the reader to the notion that developmental theory is a body of knowledge which is constantly changing and evolving. Just like the individual of any age, it has a past, a future, and a dynamic present; and the study of any one aspect will increase understanding of the others. In addition, an awareness that much of developmental theory is clinically derived—and clinically useful—may stimulate an interest in further study.

HISTORICAL OVERVIEW

Prior to the twentieth century, children were thought to be miniature adults, physically smaller, but mentally the same. This long-established pattern of thinking began to change with the work of Sigmund Freud, whose interest in childhood was peaked by the discovery of the relationship between infantile experience and adult symptomatology. For example, in the *Three Essays on the Theory of Sexuality* (1905/1968), Freud observed that

> As long ago as in the year 1896, I insisted on the significance of the years of childhood in the origin of certain important phenomena connected with sexual life, and since then I have never ceased to emphasize the part played in sexuality by the infantile factor. (p. 176)

The thought that children were sexual was shocking to Victorian Viennese—and still is today to many parents and adults. Clinicians, therefore, should not be surprised by negative adult reactions to infantile sexuality; a response based in part on the repression of their own early experience.

Freud also began to recognize maturational sequences. These eventually became the still recognized childhood developmental phases—oral, anal, Oedipal, latency, and adolescence. The idea that the mind evolves through predictable, sequential stages or phases is at the core of developmental thinking. Unfortunately, Freud did not consider adulthood from a developmental perspective; an omission which impeded the emergence of adult developmental theory for several decades.

In 1909, Freud attempted to apply his new insights to the treatment of a child, recorded in the famous case of "Little Hans." Although Freud did not actually meet with Hans, he talked about him with his father, a student, who then brought "the professor's" ideas to the boy. In his case report, Freud described the nature of infantile sexuality and Oedipal behavior—subjects that we will consider in detail in the next several chapters.

In the 1920s and 1930s, the treatment of children began, stimulated by the interest of, and rivalry between, Anna Freud and Melanie Klein (Glover, 1945). Klein's ideas, which place Oedipal phenomena in the first year of life and propose the early interpretation of unconscious content, are highly influential today in South America and in England. Anna Freud's elaboration of classical developmental theory and emphasis on the interpretation of defense before impulse are cornerstones of psychodynamic thinking and technique, particularly in the United States. As the clouds of World War II began to gather in Europe, many child therapists sought refuge in the United States where they introduced analytic concepts as they became part of the rapidly expanding child guidance movement.

As strange as it may seem today, because the idea is so completely accepted, the importance of the mother–child relationships for infant and early childhood development was not fully recognized before the 1940s and the 1950s. Then René Spitz's (1945) work on "Hospitalism" revolutionized contemporary thought. He discovered that infants who were raised in foundling homes where they received food and shelter but little in the way of love, attention, and stimulation, experienced severe developmental delays and often died before they were a year old whereas those who remained with their mothers developed normally. The study of the mother–child dyad led to an interest in the parent's contribution to childhood pathology and laid the foundation for the object relations theory which underlies much of our current understanding of normality and pathology. However, overemphasis on the parent–child interaction also produced some erroneous conclusions such as Kanner's (1943) belief that "refrigerator parents" were responsible for early infantile autism.

The Second World War provided an occasion for the study of the detrimental effects of separation and trauma upon children, resulting in the classical studies of Anna Freud and Dorothy Burlingame (Wolf, 1945) on English children who were separated from their parents for safety reasons during the London blitz.

The treatment of children, particularly in guidance clinics, became commonplace by the 1950s and led to an explosion of clinical research on development and the publication of classical books and articles, such as Berta Bornstein's (1951) paper "On Latency," Peter Blos's (1962) book *On Adolescence,* and Anna Freud's (1965) book *Normality and Pathology in Childhood.* Although countless other reference sources could be mentioned, no other publication has consistently discussed the history and evolution of developmental theory and its clinical application better than *The Psychoanalytic Study of the Child,* published yearly since 1945.

Today the developmental theory of childhood is rapidly expanding due to research in widely diverse areas. Examples may be found in the areas of infant development, fatherhood, and the biological bases of behavior. Increased knowledge of infant behavior and psychopathology has produced a new subspeciality, infant psychiatry, and created controversy over the degree of mental sophistication that is present in the mind of the infant (Dowling & Rothstein, 1989). This subject will be discussed in Chapter Three on infancy. The past decade has also seen a greatly expanded interest in the study of the relationship between fathers and their children. For a detailed consideration of this subject, the reader is referred to *Father and Child* (1982) and *Fathers and Their Families* (1989), two excellent books on the subject which were edited by Stanley Cath, Alan Gurwitt, John Munder Ross, and Linda Gunsberg.

Basic research on the biochemistry of the brain has already produced a revolution in our understanding and treatment of such psychopathological entities as manic-depressive disorder. In the near and distant future, it can be anticipated that brain research will have a similar effect on the evolution of developmental theory. Take for example the work of Kandel (1976; Kandel & Schwartz, 1982) which shows that it is possible for experience to alter the strength of neurotransmission across the synapse (the basis for memory) and produce permanent change. If life experience can alter the regulation of structures put in place genetically, then the study of the relationships between early infantile experiences and the still evolving brain may eventually produce new techniques for influencing normal and pathological development which are inconceivable at this time.

A FEW BASIC CONCEPTS

Definition of Development

The definition that I find most useful was proposed by Spitz (1965) who described it as "the emergence of forms, of function and of behavior which are the outcome of exchanges between the organism on the one hand, the inner and outer environment on the other" (p. 5). In essence, Spitz suggested that the mind evolves because of the *continuous* interactions among three sets of variables: the body (or organism) as it matures during childhood and regresses during adulthood; the mind itself (the inner environment), as it exists at any particular point in the life cycle; and external influences (the outer environment), consisting primarily of the family of origin in childhood and the family of procreation in adulthood.

As indicated by this definition, maturation and development are not the same. Maturation is a more circumscribed concept, referring to the unfolding of genetically controlled potentials, such as the abilities to walk at about 1 year of age, to read and write during the elementary school years, and to become physically and sexually mature during adolescence. All of this is encompassed in Spitz's definition by the term, *the organism.*

This definition also rejects the notion that normality or pathology may be explained by emphasizing any one set of influences over the other two. Thus, those theories which rely exclusively on either biological (current organic theories of psychopathology) or environmental (behavioral theory) influences to explain behavior will be incomplete. This definition can have great clinical relevance because it reminds diagnosticians and therapists to constantly consider biological, intrapsychic, and environmental influences as they attempt to understand and treat patients.

Children Are Different at Different Ages

If the mind and the body are constantly evolving, then it follows logically that children are different at different ages. This means that the student of development must become familiar with these differences and recognize that what is normal behavior at one age may be quite abnormal at another (see Table 1). For example, temper tantrums are to be expected at age 2 but not at age 6; phobias and nightmares are normal during the Oedipal years (ages 3–6) but not during latency (ages 6–11). Between ages 3 and 6, phobias and nightmares indicate that the child has reached the Oedipal stage of development and is engaging the issues, themes, and

Table 1. *The Stages of Development*[a]

Oral phase	0–18 months
Anal phase	1–3 years of age
Oedipal phase	3–6 years of age
Latency phase	6–12 years of age
Adolescent phase	12–20 years of age
Young adulthood	Ages 20–40
Middle adulthood	Ages 40–60
Late adulthood	Ages 60–80
Late late adulthood	Ages 80–

[a]The childhood phases were first described by Sigmund Freud; the adult stages by Erik Erikson.

conflicts which are characteristic of this phase. At age 10 the same fears, phobias, and nightmares likely indicate the presence of a neurosis.

Recognizing phase-specific behaviors allows the clinician to effectively diagnose and treat children since every aspect of the diagnostic and treatment process is based on an understanding of the child's age-related abilities to think, understand, and communicate.

The Role of the Environment

Parents are the most significant environmental force in a child's life and play an indispensable role in his or her development, particularly during infancy and early childhood. Then as the child moves out of the nuclear family into the community, environmental factors become broader based and include the influence of teachers, neighbors, peers and coaches, and the like. Recognizing the position and power of the parent is also important in considering any therapeutic intervention because children are treated only at the pleasure of their parents (see Chapter Two). Forging a therapeutic alliance with parents is facilitated by an understanding of their role in the child patient's life and by recognizing the impact that the child's problems have on the parents' adult development. Both of these subjects will be addressed repeatedly throughout this book.

The Power of Innate Forces

But parents are not the only factor influencing development and they do not by themselves determine the outcome; biological processes, sometimes referred to at a psychic level as drives or impulses, may be equally or more potent. Recognition of the power of innate forces helps the clinician understand that even when external circumstances are ideal, children will struggle and experience internal conflict—an inevitable process which is at the core of both normal and pathologic behavior—and may develop symptoms. This is particularly so when there is an imbalance between the power of the drives and the capacity of the psyche and of the environment to contain them, such as exists during the "terrible twos" and early adolescence.

AREAS OF DIFFERENCE
BETWEEN THE CHILD AND THE ADULT

In the book, *Normality and Pathology in Childhood*, which I will refer to frequently, Anna Freud (1965) described four areas of difference between children and adults. These differences are qualitative, representing aspects of the child's thinking which when misunderstood by adults can lead to inappropriate responses and frustration.

Egocentricity

The first area is *egocentricity*. During infancy

> the mothering person is not perceived by the child as having an existence of her own; she is perceived only in terms of a role assigned her within the framework of the child's needs and wishes. Accordingly, whatever happens in or to the object is understood from the aspect of satisfaction or frustration of these wishes. Every preoccupation of the mother, her concerns with other members of the family, with work or outside interests, her depressions, illnesses, absences, even her death, are transformed thereby into experiences of rejection and desertion. (A. Freud, 1945, p. 59)

This means that the infant and toddler *must* misinterpret the actions of significant adults. Under normal circumstances, these slights are compensated for by innumerable interactions of assurance and pleasure. However, when some tragedy befalls the parent/child dyad, such as the mother's death or abandonment, the sense of rejection may leave permanent emotional scars, undermining the child's emotional and intellectual development.

Under normal circumstances, the absolute egocentricity of infancy becomes relative in childhood and remains an aspect of expectation in the adult where it is tempered by cognitive maturity and comfortable control of impulses.

Immaturity of the Sexual Apparatus

The immaturity of the infantile sexual apparatus (and mental apparatus) ensures that the young child will misinterpret adult sexuality, distorting it to fit his or her physical and intellectual experience.

This accounts for parental intercourse being misunderstood as a scene of brutal violence and opens the door for all the difficulties of identifying with either the alleged victim or alleged aggressor which reveal themselves later in the growing child's uncertainty about his own sexual identity. (A. Freud, 1965, p. 59)

Consequently, children should be protected from exposure to adult sexual activity and not given detailed factual information during their early childhood. Knowledge of penetration, ejaculation, and similar adult experience by the child is often indicative of exposure to adult sexual activity or sexual abuse. This subject will be explored more thoroughly in Chapter Five.

Relative Weakness of Secondary Process Thinking

Because the young child's ability to think in logical, rational terms is limited, he or she will understand the world differently from adults and will misinterpret many events. Parents and therapists who understand this concept will not become frustrated when young children cling to misperceptions and react in seemingly inappropriate ways. For example, I was asked to do an emergency consultation on a pediatric ward for a 4-year-old boy who had been admitted with a broken arm. Upon awakening from surgery, he had begun to cry and could not be consoled. As we began to talk about why he was crying, he told me that his arm was gone and he wanted it back. He could not see his arm inside the cast which covered it and assumed that it was gone. After he and I bandaged, removed, and rebandaged a cast placed on the arm of a doll, he began to calm down, having grasped the idea that his own arm was "safe" inside the cast.

The Different Sense of Time

Because the mind of the young child is undeveloped, there is little ability to tolerate frustration and delay gratification. This instant need for gratification of wishes and cognitive immaturity ensures that the young child will experience time differently than will adults (Colarusso, 1979; 1988).

It is these latter factors which will decide whether the intervals set for feeding, the absence of the mother, the duration of nursery attendance, of hospitalization, etc. will seem to the child short or long, tolerable or intolerable, and as a result will prove harmless or harmful in their consequences. (A. Freud, 1965, pp. 60–61)

Clinicians are often asked to give opinions on all of the situations described in the Anna Freud quote. An understanding of the child's different sense of time will allow the clinician to make recommendations which take the child's needs into account, but which often frustrate parents and other caregivers who resent the restrictions placed upon their freedom to use time for their own purposes.

These basic differences between the adult and the child directly affect their respective experiences in therapy. Whereas the adult patient willingly enters treatment to achieve greater success in work or better sexual relationships, the child patient resents "having to adapt to an unpalpable reality and to give up immediate wish fulfillments and secondary gains" (A. Freud, 1965, p. 27). The adult's tendency to repeat, which is an important component of transference, is in contradistinction to the child's hunger for new experiences and relationships. The adult's willingness to work through is countered by the child's age-appropriate use of opposite defense mechanisms, such as denial, isolation, and projection. The strongest ally which the child therapist has is a developmental one, the desire of the child to grow up, to imitate and emulate older children and adults.

REGRESSION AS A NORMAL PHENOMENON IN CHILD DEVELOPMENT

Regression, the abandonment of recently acquired functions and abilities and their substitution with forms, functions, and behaviors from earlier periods, is a ubiquitous phenomenon in childhood. In the course of normal development, the regressions which occur are temporary and self-limiting, usually related to some identifiable stress, such as fatigue, illness, or parental absence, or facing a new expectation or developmental task, such as going to school or dating. When pathological processes dominate, the regressions are more pronounced, last longer, and involve more mental functions and behaviors, sometimes resulting in a sense of permanence called *fixation*.

Anna Freud (1965) suggested that "backward moves" (p. 98) accompany all important achievements in childhood, including control of motility, reality testing, bowel and bladder control, the mastery of anxiety, frustration tolerance, language acquisition, and superego functioning. The capacity to attain a higher level of functioning is no guarantee that such performance will be stable or continuous.

> On the contrary: occasional returns to more infantile behavior have to be taken as a normal sign. Thus, nonsense talk or even babbling have a rightful place in the child's life, alongside rational speech and alternating with it. Clean toilet habits are not acquired at one go, but take the long back-and-forth way

through an interminable series of successes, relapses and accidents. (A. Freud, 1965, p. 99)

In fact, this back-and-forth, gradual progression is to be preferred to "instantaneous change-over" and sudden "transformations."

> But convenient as such transformations may be for the child's environment, the diagnostician views them with suspicion and ascribes them not to the ordinary flow of progressive development but to traumatic influences and anxieties which unduly hasten its normal course. According to experience, the slow method of trial and error, progression and temporary reversal is more appropriate to healthier psychic growth. (p. 99)

THE CONCEPT OF DEVELOPMENT LINES

In *Normality and Pathology in Childhood* (1965), Anna Freud also introduced a concept for tracing circumscribed aspects of development *across* developmental phases, introducing the term *developmental lines*. Their use as a description of the basic interaction between the ego and the id at various developmental levels enables the clinician to conceptualize normal and pathological processes and enhances the ability to communicate information to parents.

Among the developmental lines described by Anna Freud are "From Dependency to Emotional Self-Reliance and Adult Object Relationships" (pp. 64–68), "From Suckling to Rational Eating" (pp. 69–72) and "From Egocentricity to Companionship" (p. 78). Building on this concept, Robert Nemiroff and myself (1981) introduced the concept of *adult developmental lines*, thus continuing the description of various aspects of development from childhood through adulthood. The conceptualization of developmental lines will be utilized throughout this book. A good example of its use in childhood may be found in Chapter Four (p. 58), where the developmental line of "From Wetting and Soiling to Bladder and Bowel Control" is used as a rationale for understanding the intrapsychic consequences of toilet training.

With this brief introduction to the subject of child development, let us turn our attention to the diagnostic process in childhood and then to the first two decades of life, considering in chronological order the oral, anal, Oedipal, latency and adolescent phases of development.

CHAPTER 2

The Diagnostic Process with Children

INTRODUCTION

This chapter describes some of the techniques used in an in-depth psychiatric evaluation of a child, and provides rationales for their use. A thorough evaluation enables the diagnostician to understand the biological, intrapsychic, and environmental factors that have produced the existing symptom complex, to make a diagnosis, and to formulate a practical treatment plan that will be of the greatest benefit to the child and his or her family.

The procedures involved differ somewhat from those used in the evaluation of adults because of the *developmental differences* between the two. Already discussed in Chapter One, these differences affect the diagnostic process as follows:

1. The immaturity of the child's mind does not allow him or her to understand the need for an evaluation or to participate in it with the same degree of comprehension or cooperation as the adult.
2. Children are not independent. They live with parents or other adults who control many aspects of their lives—and the diagnostic evaluation. Parents or other caretakers not only bring the child for help, but also provide information about the present and past which the child cannot give because of a lack of knowledge and intellectual immaturity.
3. Since the developmental process is continually unfolding and children are different at different ages, techniques and procedures will vary depending upon the developmental level of the child.

For example, the evaluation of an Oedipal-aged child will be significantly different from that of an adolescent.

The component parts of a diagnostic evaluation are:

1. A history obtained from the child's parents or other caretakers and additional relevant sources, such as physicians and teachers.
2. Diagnostic interviews with the child.
3. Additional procedures, such as psychological, neurological, or educational testing.
4. Diagnostic impressions.
5. Treatment planning.
6. A summary conference in which the findings of the diagnostic process are presented.

EVALUATION PROCEDURES FOR YOUNG CHILDREN

Although the component parts are the same in the evaluation of younger children and adolescents, they are not utilized in the same manner because of the developmental differences between the two. For children from birth through latency (approximately 11 or 12 years of age) the sequence of the evaluation is as follows:

1. The initial contact—almost always made by a parent or other caretaker.
2. The history—usually obtained in three or four 45-minute sessions with the parents alone.
3. The diagnostic interviews with the child—at least two 45-minute sessions with the child alone.
4. Additional procedures—obtained at this point, if needed, after assessing the data collected during the history taking and diagnostic interviews.
5. Diagnostic and treatment formulations by the diagnostician.
6. A summary conference with the parents but not with the child.

The initial contact. The initial contact may be made in person or by telephone. In either event, it is essential to remember that in most instances the decision to seek professional assistance was made with considerable apprehension, fear, and misgiving. For the parent, who sees the child as both a responsibility and an extension of him or herself, the expected response is criticism for real or imagined wrongdoing. The very act of seeking help is often accompanied by considerable guilt. For the child, depending upon age, the mental health professional may be simply another powerful adult, a sinister stranger, or, in the case of an adolescent, a source of apprehension or shame. A warm, friendly telephone voice or a pleasant greeting accompanied by a handshake and sensitivity to the above-mentioned feelings will diminish apprehension and lay the foundation for a productive diagnostic process.

In the evaluation of young children, the initial contact is inevitably made with an adult since children rarely recognize the need for treatment and are not capable of assuming responsibility for participation in the evaluation process.

The history. The history is taken from the parents because the child is not able to describe current problems or past experience in an organized manner. This information is gathered before seeing the child because it assists the diagnostician in understanding the child's communications which are often in the form of play or incomplete verbalizations. The division of the history into (1) identifying information, chief complaint, and history of the present illness, (2) developmental history, and (3) parental history will be considered shortly.

Diagnostic interview with the child. Once the child separates from the parent and is comfortable in the playroom, he or she will communicate through actions and words. An understanding of developmental theory and knowledge of the individual child allows the diagnostician to assess normality and pathology as the interviews progress. The need to collect diagnostic information from psychological and educational testing, or from medical procedures can only be determined after the presenting problems have been described during the history-taking and diagnostic interviews. Since ancillary procedures subject the child to anxiety-producing situations and may involve additional expense, they should only be ordered when the information they provide is essential to obtaining a clear diagnostic impression.

Formulating the diagnostic impression and treatment plan. Once the necessary data are collected, the hard work begins. Although the process of formulating a diagnostic impression begins with the initial contact, it cannot be completed in a responsible manner without a thorough consideration of all the data from the history, interviews, and ancillary procedures. The formulation of a descriptive, dynamic, and developmental diagnosis is followed by treatment recommendations which are based on the diagnoses and the realities of the patient's life.

The summary conference. Following the completion of the evaluation of a younger child, a conference is held with the parents during which the findings are presented in detail. The child is not present because he or she would not be able to fully understand the concepts being presented and might experience unnecessary anxiety from exposure to the information itself or parental comments and reactions to it. In preparation for the summary conference, the diagnostician should organize the findings and consider how he or she wants to present them to the parents to ensure clarity and comfort. An organized presentation, usually from prepared notes, indicates to the parents that their concerns have been taken seriously and were thoroughly considered. Such an approach is important because the decision to accept the treatment recommendations will be made by the parents, not the child. In addition to serving its diagnostic function, the evaluation period allows the parents time to form a relationship with the person—at first a stranger—to whom they may entrust the care of their child. Many cases are lost before they begin because a rapport has not been established between the parents and the potential therapist.

EVALUATION PROCEDURES WITH ADOLESCENTS

The diagnostic process with an adolescent differs from a younger child because of the developmental differences between the two. In conducting an evaluation of an adolescent patient, it is important to keep in mind the following:

1. The adolescent is in the process of psychologically separating from his or her parents and wants to be treated and thought of as an individual.
2. Because of the upsurge of sexual feelings generated by puberty, adolescents are unable to enter comfortably into a close, open relationship with others, particularly adults.
3. The adolescent is capable of understanding the complexities of the diagnostic process and of participating in an active manner. He or she can provide historical information, describe internal states and external circumstances without assistance from parents. Furthermore, he or she is able to understand the diagnostic findings and treatment recommendations and to participate in the decision-making process about their acceptance or rejection. For these reasons, the sequence of the evaluation differs from the one used with younger children.

The *initial telephone contact* is still usually made by a parent. After listening to the parent's concerns and outlining the diagnostic process, the clinician should attempt to schedule the diagnostic interviews directly with the adolescent. Parents are often relieved by this suggestion because of the anticipation of a battle with the adolescent over scheduling.

The *diagnostic interviews* with the adolescent are held first in order to convey the following message: "I respect you as an individual and want to learn what I need to know about you first hand. I recognize your burgeoning independence and ability to participate in this diagnostic process."

The *history-taking interviews* with the parents follow and serve the same functions as they do with younger children. If required, additional data are obtained from *ancillary procedures*.

Diagnostic and treatment formulations are then made.

Two *summary conferences* are held: the first with the adolescent alone, the second with his or her parents. This sequence conveys a strong message of respect for the adolescent and increases the chances that the patient may accept the recommendations made. It also permits the adolescent to know, in advance, what his or her parents will be told and to discuss any objections with the diagnostician. The parent conference should follow as quickly as possible, ideally on the same day. Adolescent and parents are then asked to discuss the recommendations together and arrive at a course of action.

Obviously these guidelines may need to be altered from time to time depending on circumstances, diagnosis, and other factors. For instance, one would operate differently in a true emergency (rare in child psychiatry) or in the evaluation of a severely retarded or psychotic youngster. Furthermore, these guidelines will not prepare one for those unusual situations which will inevitably arise. In all instances, common sense, a thorough understanding of the developmental process, and sensitivity and empathy should determine one's action.

COLLECTING AND RECORDING THE DATA

Collecting and recording the diagnostic data are two different but interrelated processes. An understanding of diagnostic procedures and developmental theory provides a rationale for each step, ensuring that all necessary information will be gathered in as sensitive and efficient a manner as possible.

Depending upon need, the collected information may remain in raw form or be organized for verbal or written presentation. The following outline is intended as a guide which includes techniques for collecting and organizing the data. An example of a completed evaluation concludes this chapter.

The identifying information may be organized as follows:

Identifying Information

1. Father's full name, age, occupation, description
2. Mother's full name, age, occupation, description
3. Children, in chronological order, full name, birthdates, school and grade, description
4. Others living in the home—full name, age, reason for presence in the home

The identifying information provides the basic realities of the child's life and a skeletal framework on which to build an understanding of his or her problems. Symptoms and development will be influenced by the presence or absence of parents and siblings, socioeconomic status, and other life circumstances. Be sure to note whether or not the child is adopted and the relationship of the child to parents and siblings, biological, step, or foster. Birthdates are more useful than age in years because they allow for a more accurate chronology of the relationships among symptoms, life events, and developmental sequences.

Parents provide this information in the evaluation of younger children. Collect it from the adolescent and his or her parents, looking for differences in attitude and emphasis.

Referral Source

Briefly describe the source of the referral and the process involved. This helps determine whether the child is seen as a problem within the home and/or outside of it. Recording these data also serves as a reminder to express thanks to the referral source and to convey information about the findings of the evaluation to those individuals or institutions (such as the school) who may be of assistance to the child.

Chief Complaint

The chief complaint should be elicited from, and described in (1) the child's words, (2) the parent's words, and (3) the words of other referring agencies such as the school or pediatrician.

It is not unusual for the chief complaint to vary enormously because of the different understanding and concerns of the child, the parents, and the referring agency.

The chief complaint(s) should be recorded in a phrase or sentence: "He wets the bed." "He's unmanageable." "She disturbs the other children in the classroom."

History of the Present Illness

The initial interview with the parents usually concerns itself with the history of the present illness. Parents should be encouraged to convey their concerns in a manner of their choosing. This allows them to control the flow of information, thus allaying any anxiety about being embarrassed by the diagnostician's questions or forced to reveal sensitive details before they are ready to do so. Such a technique conveys a sense of respect for feelings and defenses and emphasizes the importance placed on the parent's impressions and concerns by the diagnostician.

A similar procedure is followed with adolescents but the diagnostician should be prepared to take a more active role if the patient has difficulty or is hesitant to describe his or her concerns.

After the patient or parents have had the opportunity to tell their story, proceed to ask those additional questions which will provide you with a detailed understanding of the presenting problems.

In recording this information for written or verbal presentation, *each* symptom should be described (1) clearly and concisely, (2) chronologically, particularly in relationship to major developmental themes, and (3) in terms of what external influences increase or decrease the severity of the phenomenon.

Developmental History

In taking a developmental history, we utilize our knowledge of normal and pathological processes to gain a detailed understanding of the patient's past in order to relate past experience to symptom formation and to interferences with normal developmental progression in the present and future. Through the developmental history, we come to understand the uniqueness of each patient's journey through life. Consequently, our diagnostic impressions will be more than vague generalizations which could apply to anyone in the same diagnostic category and our treatment recommendations will address specific needs.

The outline of the information to be gathered which follows is a distillation of the development theory of childhood, presented in this form to help the diagnostician collect and present the data in an organized manner.

Some of the developmental information involved will be provided spontaneously by the parents or child. The rest is gathered by asking questions in a more systematic fashion than was used to collect the history of the present illness. Ask the parents to bring baby books, pictures, report cards, and other source material which may help them remember details, particularly about infancy and early childhood. Adolescents are quite capable of giving a developmental history of latency and adolescence, but they, like most individuals, rarely remember much about the first 5 or 6 years of life because of the blanket repression which occurs at the end of the Oedipal stage of development.

The Pregnancy, Labor, and Delivery. (1) Was this pregnancy planned or unplanned? (2) Were there any previous pregnancies and/or births? (3) Were there problems with the pregnancy? Did the mother have any illnesses or complications? Did she abuse drugs or alcohol? (4) How much weight did she gain (normally, about twenty pounds)? (5) What was the psychological health of each parent? (6) Did the parents have a gender preference? (7) What was the nature of the parents relationship with each other? (8) How long was the labor (approximately 12–14 hours for the first pregnancy, less thereafter)? (9) Were there any complications? (10) Was the labor spontaneous or induced? (11) Was the presentation vertex (head first) or breech (greater incidence of complications)? (12) Was the delivery vaginal or Caesarean? Was it uncomplicated? (13) What was the baby's condition at the time of birth? (14) Was the baby examined by a pediatrician? (15) Was the father present during the labor and delivery? (16) How was the child's name chosen?

The First Year of Life (the Oral Phase). (1) Were the parents psychologically ready to care for the child? (2) How much time did they devote to parenting? (3) What was the quality of their parenting? Of their relationship to each other? (4) Was the baby breast- or bottle-fed? Was he or she a strong sucker? (5) When did the baby begin to adjust to the 24-hour day–night cycle (sleeping for longer periods at night by 6 weeks of age)? (6) What was the baby's temperament? (7) When did the smile response occur (by 3 months of age)? (8) Was thumb-sucking prominent? Was a pacifier used? (9) When did weaning occur? (10) Did the child have any major illnesses or operations (at any time in childhood or adolescence)?

Ages 1–3 (the Anal Phase). (1) When did language develop (single words by 1 year, short sentences by age 2)? (2) Describe gross and fine motor development (running by age 2; using pencils and crayons and climbing steps by age 3). (3) Were there any prolonged (more than several days) separations from the parents? (4) Did the child gradually move away, physically and psychologically from the primary caretakers? (5) Was object constancy achieved by age 3? (6) When was toilet training begun? How was it managed? (7) To what extent were negativism and other aspects of the "terrible twos" present? (7) Were the parents able to set limits in an empathetic, consistent manner?

Ages 3–6 (the Oedipal Phase). (1) What was the child's attitude toward the parent of the same sex? of the opposite sex? (2) Was the child sexually curious? Was masturbation observed? (3) What was the child's attitude about being a boy or a girl? (4) How did the parents respond to the child's Oedipal strivings? Were they seductive? Were they punitive or restrictive? (5) Were signs of the infantile neurosis noted? (6) What was the nature of the child's first experiences at school? Did he or she separate easily from parents? Relate to teachers and peers? Possess the perceptual maturity necessary for formal learning?

Ages 6–11 (Latency). (1) Was the child ready to comfortably move out of the nuclear family into the community? (2) In regard to elementary school, how did the child function academically? How did he or she get along with teachers? Was the child accepted by his peers, particularly of the same sex? (3) Was there evidence of conscience formation? Did the child demonstrate increased control of fantasy and behavior? An ability to accept rules and limitations in play and social settings? (4) Was a strong sexual identification with same sex peers and adults evident? (5) Did physical maturation and increased intellectual abilities lead to the emergence of athletic, artistic, and social skills and hobbies?

Ages 11–20 (Adolescence). (1) When did puberty occur? What was the adolescent's reaction? Was he or she prepared? (2) Was there gradual evidence in early adolescence of acceptance of the physically mature body? (3) Was there evidence of mood swings, inconsistent behavior, and regression—external evidences that intrapsychic change was underway? (4) Was the second individuation, the physical and psychological separation from parents, gradually occurring? (5) Were peers becoming an increasingly important part of the adolescent's life? What was the nature of peer relationships? (6) Did integration of the sexually mature body lead to dating in midadolescence and the beginning of a sexual life by late adolescence? (7) What was the adolescent's attitude toward homosexual thoughts, feelings, and actions? (8) In junior and senior high school how did the adolescent achieve academically? Get along with teachers? Plan for work or further schooling? (9) Was the ability to think abstractly evident and growing? What were the adolescent's attitudes toward social, moral, and religious values?

A similar consideration of the questions to be asked about the phases of development in adulthood will be presented in Chapter Nine, The Adult Developmental Diagnostic Process.

Parental History

A brief history of the parent's major childhood and adult experiences and current life should be obtained because of the relationship between past experience and current child-rearing practices. The information volunteered is often extremely relevant to understanding the child's symptoms. For example:

"I wet the bed until I was nine, just like Joan."
or
"My mother died when I was pregnant with Tom. God took away one life and gave me another."

Both parents should be involved in the diagnostic process if at all possible. Insist on interviewing both parents, determining whether more information will be obtained by seeing them together and/or individually. Many clinicians avoid dealing with assertive or difficult parents, particularly fathers, because of fear and anxiety. Frequently this is due to an unconscious identification with the child and their position of vulnerability to parental power and control.

Diagnostic Interviews

Parents often need help in preparing their child for these interviews. There are two essential points to be considered. First, the child should be told in advance that he or she will be coming to see you. Very young children should be given 2 or 3 days notice. Latency-aged youngsters should be informed up to a week in advance. Adolescents should be told about the nature of your meetings with them during the initial telephone contact when the appointments are arranged.

Second, parents should be encouraged to tell the truth simply and straightforwardly about what will happen during the interviews. Since parents tend to avoid this task out of fear of alarming the child or encountering resistance, be sure to ask the child at the beginning of the first diagnostic session what he or she has been told about your meeting.

When interviewing a young patient, advise the parents in advance that you will concentrate your attention on the child and discourage them from giving you additional information or asking questions in front of the child. After being introduced, greet your patient warmly and assess the child's level of anxiety and ability to separate. In very young children, and others with marked separation problems, it may be necessary to ask the parent to accompany you to the playroom and remain until the child is comfortable enough for the parent to leave.

Once in the playroom, let the child determine the course of the interview. Some children will immediately begin to play, while others will sit and wait for directions. Depending on their age and issues, adolescents may come to the first interview alone or accompanied by a parent. In either event, an attitude of respect and a warm handshake will allay anxiety and encourage cooperation.

Remember that the purpose of these interviews is diagnostic. That means your aim is to gain as much information as you can about the patient's personality structure and problems in an unobtrusive manner. Children reveal themselves through play and words. Adolescents usually prefer to talk. Many children and adolescents will not discuss their symptoms with you directly, and it is not always advisable or necessary to ask directly about them. With experience and an increased knowledge of child development and psychopathology, it becomes increasingly easy to assess the derivative material that the patient must inevitably present through play and words. Interpretation has little, if any, place in a diagnostic interview.

During the course of the interviews, you should perform a mental status examination, assessing the following areas:

1. *Appearance and behavior*—Observe the child's height, weight, and build. Look for unusual body movements or mannerisms, level of physical activity, and style of dress.

2. *Characteristics of speech*—Note the rate, rhythm, and clarity of the child's speech. Assess the size and age-appropriateness of vocabulary and any speech impediments.

3. *Affect*—What is the predominant feeling tone? Are the affects present appropriate to the thought content? Can the child express affects verbally in an age-appropriate manner?

4. *Object relations*—Does the patient have a clear sense of self and other? What is the level of his or her ability to relate to you?

5. *Thinking*—Assess the age-appropriateness of reality testing and secondary process thinking. Explore the nature and content of fantasies and daydreams, prominent defenses, and persistent or overdetermined themes.

6. *Intelligence*—Estimate the child's level of intelligence by observing his or her vocabulary, fund of knowledge, and motor skills.

7. *Orientation*—Is the patient oriented as to time, person, and place?

8. *Capacity for insight*—What is the patient's ability to think introspectively? To observe and examine his or her thoughts and actions?

9. *Motivation*—Observe the patient's desire to rid himself or herself

of painful thoughts, feelings, and actions. Consider his or her ability to discuss problems or demonstrate them through play.

Ancillary Procedures

Any data obtained from psychological or educational testing, or from examinations performed by physicians or other professionals should be recorded here.

Review of Records

Records of any kind which have diagnostic significance may be summarized and recorded at this point.

Diagnosis

It is in the formulation of the diagnosis and treatment plan that a detailed understanding of the patient is translated into concepts which may be meaningfully communicated to others. In its most complete form, the diagnostic impression should be expressed in three ways: descriptively, dynamically, and developmentally.

1. *Descriptive diagnosis.* The most widely used descriptive system of diagnosis is contained in the current edition of the *Diagnostic and Statistical Manual of Mental Disorders* published by the American Psychiatric Association. Because this system does not provide a picture of the patient's intrapsychic life or of his or her development, dynamic and developmental diagnoses are added.

2. *Dynamic diagnosis.* The patient's symptoms are explained in terms of intrapsychic conflict, impulse, and defense, utilizing Freud's topographical (conscious and unconscious) and structural (id, ego, and superego) theories.

3. *Developmental diagnosis.* The patient's life experience at each developmental phase is utilized to understand the normal and pathological aspects of his or her personality. Symptoms are traced across developmental phases and described in terms of their effect on the engagement of phase-specific, developmental tasks.

Treatment Recommendations

Treatment recommendations should be detailed and specific, tailored to the patient's pathology and individual circumstances. When based on the large fund of information gathered in a thorough diagnostic process such as the one just described, the recommended interventions are more likely to be presented to the parents and to the child or adolescent in a manner which increases the likelihood of their acceptance.

Summary Conference

Your patients are entitled to an organized, prepared, summation of their problems and your recommendations. What you tell them should be presented in a manner which they can understand, free of jargon; thus facilitating their ability to make an informed decision on your comments. It is important to be honest and kind, but not to the point that you fail to present a realistic picture of the patient's problems and treatment requirements.

Obviously, your language and manner will be determined by who you are addressing. For example, you would speak differently to an adolescent than to his parents.

In nearly all instances, it is wise to suggest that your recommendations be discussed and considered at the patient's home, over a few days. Those patients who rush into treatment, or who are persuaded to make an immediate decision to begin, often drop out at some point in time—which is a frustrating and painful experience for patient and therapist alike. Suggest that your prospective adolescent patient and his or her parents discuss your recommendations together and then inform you of their decision.

When approached in the manner described, your completed evaluation should give you a clear understanding of the patient; establish a relationship of respect and understanding between you and the potential patient and his or her family—the basis of a therapeutic alliance; and enhance the chances that your recommendations will be accepted and effective.

CASE REPORT

This report of a diagnostic evaluation of a 9-year-old boy is based on the data gathered during four interviews with both parents, two diagnostic sessions with the patient, and the psychological testing.

1. Identifying information:
   (a) Father—George, 37, a tall, thin, quiet pharmacist.
   (b) Mother—Louise, 35, a slightly overweight, loving but anxious housewife.
   (c) Jim, the patient, born July 5, 1976. A stocky, energetic 9-year-old, he was in the fourth grade when the evaluation began.

    (d) Harold, his natural brother, born August 14, 1980; an out-
going, friendly first grader.

    (e) Carol, born December 7, 1982, Jim's natural sister. She was in
nursery school, doing well, but experiencing some separation
difficulties.

2. Referral source:

Mother brought Jim for evaluation after discussion with her therapist, who was also a child psychiatrist.

3. Chief complaint(s):

    (a) Parents—"He can't be satisfied or comforted . . . he has tem-
per tantrums and is very selfish. He can't keep friends."

    (b) Jim—"My parents don't listen to me. They prefer my brother
over me . . . . Sometimes I think there are rattlesnakes in my bed."

4. History of the present illness:

Jim's unhappiness, which began in the first grade and seemed to be
self-generated, was expressed in concerns that his parents didn't understand or like him and preferred his brother. "He can't be satisfied or
comforted," said his mother. His temper tantrums had been occurring
since age 2; they usually followed episodes in which Jim felt neglected or
abused. For example, while Jim was talking on the phone, someone in the
family made a noise. He screamed, shouted, banged the table, and threw
a book. On another occasion he threw himself on the floor and screamed.
The difficulty with friends appeared to result from attempts to control the
relationships with other boys or a need to avoid them entirely.

A phobia was described by Jim but not by his parents. He had
nightmares a few times a month and was concerned that rattlesnakes
were in his bed. Jim knew they were not really there, but wondered if the
snakes might be invisible. His fears led to mild obsessional preoccupations that sometimes made it difficult for him to get to sleep.

5. Developmental history:

Jim was a planned child, the product of an uneventful pregnancy
and delivery. During infancy the mother–child relationship was close and
constant. Mother felt that the problems precipitating her own treatment
had little to do with Jim and did not interfere with her desire or ability
to love and take care of him. "He was a good baby, healthy and calm. I
particularly loved to feed him. He was so responsive at those times."

Jim was weaned by 18 months, except for a bedtime bottle which he
demanded until he was 2½ years old. Bowel and bladder control were
achieved by age 3. In all likelihood toilet training was accompanied by
occasional outbursts of anger and frustration from both parents, generated by Jim's negativism and refusal to comply. Mother would back
down and give in; father would become more rigid. In essence, their

respective attitudes toward Jim's impulses continued throughout the Oedipal phase and latency. There were no prolonged parent–child separations during the first 3 years of life. Jim became increasingly assertive, insisting on doing things his way. By age 3, he had developed a strong sense of self.

Historical data from the Oedipal phase, ages 3 to 6, was difficult to obtain because of the striking degree of anxiety present in both parents when questions were posed about these years. However, they did recall that between 4 and 6 years of age Jim worried that rattlesnakes might be in the house. He asked many sexual questions which were usually answered in great detail. His parents observed his masturbating frequently. One day at dinner, the father casually told Jim to eat so he would grow big and strong. A few minutes later, Jim proudly displayed his erection, saying it was growing big and strong, too. Father responded by telling Jim to go to his room if he wanted to masturbate. During those years Jim clearly preferred his mother and particularly enjoyed opportunities to crawl into bed with her or watch her dress. His parents maintained an "open door policy," that is, free access to the parental bedroom and to the bathroom.

In school Jim was moderately successful academically but had mild difficulty sitting still and finishing his work. He did not keep friends very long because of his demanding ways and immaturity.

6. Parental history:

Jim's father was an only child. Raised in an intact family, his childhood was characterized by shyness and studiousness. A reserved man, he was very disturbed by Jim's brashness and temper tantrums. He appeared to be inhibited and in need of treatment himself.

Jim's mother was the youngest of four children. Her parents had a troubled marriage but remained together. She described her childhood as unhappy. Like Jim, she felt neglected and misunderstood by her parents. She went into therapy to deal with her anxiety and low self-esteem.

7. Diagnostic interviews:

Jim's parents were encouraged to tell their son why he was being brought to see me and to be prepared to answer any questions he might have about the office setting, the length of the interview, and so forth. It was suggested that he be told several days in advance of the interview to allow him time to consider the idea and form any questions and concerns. The father would bring Jim to the interview; he was asked to make the introduction and then to wait for Jim in the waiting room.

After the introduction, Jim bounded into the office and sat on the couch. Obviously nervous, he paused a moment to take in the surroundings before beginning. "I wanted to see if you were like the psychiatrists on TV. You're not; you're not bald and fat." I was struck by the anxiety, openness, and desire to relate in this bright, engaging child. Without prompting, Jim began to talk of his worries; his father had encouraged him to do so. He had known what psychiatrists do anyway and he agreed with his parents that he was unhappy. When I asked about the reasons for his unhappiness, Jim replied that his parents favored his younger brother. He was blamed for things his brother did. The intensity of Jim's feelings and his excellent verbal abilities were increasingly obvious. Later, after complaining that his parents did not pay enough attention to him, Jim looked me straight in the eye, pleading for understanding and acceptance. "I don't think adults understand how kids think," he said. Here was a child in considerable pain, eager for understanding and help. When asked about other worries, Jim replied that he could not get people to do what he wanted them to do. That morning his brother and a friend had messed up his bedroom. He yelled to his mother to come and help. All she did was yell at him for yelling. As Jim talked, his considerable problems in peer relationships became obvious.

"Can you tell me about your dreams?" I asked.

"Well, I don't have many anymore," he replied. "But I worry about going to bed. I saw a movie about snakes and now I'm afraid there are rattlesnakes in my bed." He explained how he lifted the covers before getting into bed to be sure that it was safe. "Maybe somebody sneaks in my room and sprays the snakes with invisible spray. I sleep with my legs up just to be sure." I was impressed by Jim's readiness to reveal his thoughts and by the revelation of the phobia, a symptom unrecognized by his parents.

Near the end of the interview I explained the steps in the evaluation and the need for psychological testing. Jim readily agreed to go and eagerly accepted the invitation to return for a second diagnostic interview.

The second interview was much like the first. Jim seemed less anxious. He continued to express resentment at his parents and brother, at anyone who did not do things his way. Noting the absence of any play, I invited Jim into the playroom which adjoined the office. After surveying the toys, Jim decided to draw. Over the next 20 minutes he obsessively drew a monster. When asked to tell about the monster, he revealed this fantasy: "He lives alone. People don't like him. He goes out and gets food and comes back. Maybe he'll get a friend someday." The lonely monster was understood to represent Jim's feelings about himself—ugly and isolated.

8. Mental status examination:

Jim was a bright, stocky, active, latency-aged boy who expressed himself easily, sometimes with passion. Affect, which ranged from happiness to anger, was appropriate to thought content. Thinking was logical, goal directed, and age appropriate. Jim had considerable access to his fantasies. His ego was strong and intact. His intelligence was estimated to be above average or superior, partly because of Jim's unusual capacity for a boy of his age to describe his thoughts and feelings. He was curious and introspective, indicating that he would work well in therapy.

9. Additional procedures:

Psychological testing, which was ordered to assess the strength of Jim's ego and his intelligence and to further elaborate information about his fantasies, provided the following information:

> In summary, this boy presents the picture of an anxiety neurosis, fueled by Oedipal conflicts and a prominent sense of castratedness, but underlaid with conscious pregenital conflicts (oral-dependent and oral-aggressive), such that he typically experiences the call to appropriate competitiveness and sharing as a call to battle, with a resultant regression in adaptive and defensive (obsessional) ego functions and modes of object relatedness (he becomes increasingly infantile) as depressive feelings come to the fore.

On the Wechsler Intelligence Scale for Children (WISC) his Verbal I.Q. was 118–125; Performance I.Q., 100–113; Total I.Q., 110–121. There was "a developing characterological preference for acting reasonably and rationally, and thinking things through before acting on them . . . . His depression seems related to guilt over his competitive-aggressive wishes."

10. Review of records:

There were no records of significance to be reviewed.

11. Diagnosis:

A. *Descriptive diagnosis.* Axis I—Although the patient's symptomatology satisfied some of the criteria for Oppositional Defiant Disorder (313.81), Dysthymia (300.40), and Simple Phobia (300.29), none of these DSM-III-R diagnoses adequately described his pathology.

Axis II—none

Axis III—none

Axis IV—Code 2, Mild

Axis V—65, Mild to moderate symptoms

B. *Dynamic diagnosis.* Jim's low-frustration tolerance, as demonstrated by his self-centeredness and temper tantrums, indicated significant problems with impulse control. His ego and superego, relatively intact and functional in most areas, were unable to modulate and control the strong aggressive impulses which broke through at the slightest sign of frustration. Despite the problems with impulse control and the tendency to regress easily, Jim was thought to be psychologically intact, struggling primarily with Oedipal conflicts. The failure to resolve these conflicts has resulted in the formation of neurotic symptoms, that is, anxiety, obsessional tendencies, and a phobia about rattlesnakes.

C. *Developmental diagnosis.* Jim was born into an intact, loving family. Steady developmental progression was noted during infancy because of consistent loving care and the absence of major illness. The anal phase was characterized by continued progression in most areas, but clear evidence of difficulty on the part of both parents in setting limits. Weaning was not fully accomplished until 2½ years of age, and the normal negativism of the toddler was reacted to by avoidance and/or rigidity, thus limiting Jim's ability to develop the capacity to regulate and control powerful impulses, such as anger.

As evidenced by Jim's preference for his mother, his masturbation and his sexual curiosity, it was clear that he had reached the Oedipal phase of development and became immersed in the sexual and aggressive issues central to it. The anxious inability of the parents to recall many factual details about these years and their unconsciously seductive practices, such as consistently allowing Jim to sleep with them and observing them undressed, suggested that he was overstimulated sexually. His failure to resolve Oedipal conflicts and issues had led to the presence of neurotic symptomatology and the failure to act like a normal latency-aged boy.

12 and 13. Treatment recommendations and summary conference:

Conclusions: Because his psychopathology was primarily neurotic, Jim was considered an excellent candidate for child analysis. The operating diagnosis was a psychoneurosis, anxiety type, with phobic and obsessional features. Pregenital components were represented by the temper tantrums and self-centeredness. Jim was bright, verbal, eager for help, and clearly aware of his problems. Equally important, his parents were stable, psychologically minded, and able to support the treatment.

During the summary conference the nature of Jim's psychopathology and the recommendation for child analysis was presented to his parents. They were encouraged to consider the matter seriously and to feel free to ask any questions. Four days later they called, announcing their decision to begin the analysis.

Jim was seen 4 times a week. Parental conferences were held weekly during the opening phase and approximately twice a month thereafter. Both parents provided excellent support throughout the analysis, bringing Jim regularly for sessions, observing his behavior, and considering their own interactions with him.

A detailed description of the treatment process of this case and two discussions by Jules Glenn M.D. and Isidor Bernstein, M.D. are contained in a recently published book entitled *Psychoanalytic Case Studies* (1991) edited by G. Pirooz Sholevar M.D. and Jules Glenn, M.D. (see Colarusso, 1991). A thirteen-year follow-up will be presented in Chapter Ten, Young Adulthood.

CHAPTER 3

The Oral Phase (Ages 0–1)

Infancy, or the oral phase in Freud's terminology, covers the first 12 to 18 months of life. This period of intense growth and development is currently the subject of great interest by researchers and clinicians alike, resulting in significant advances in knowledge and major theoretical change and controversy. The controversy arises in part because infancy is a preverbal phase, and thus our assumptions about mental activity during this time cannot be validated by the infant. This is the only phase of development in which this is true. By contrast, much of our knowledge of childhood, which was initially obtained from work with adults, was later confirmed (or refuted) by the direct observation and treatment of children who were able to tell us what they were thinking.

HISTORICAL CONSIDERATIONS

Many years ago, Edward Glover (1945) insisted that our conceptualizations of infancy must be based on *plausibility*. He was speaking in the midst of the controversy between Anna Freud and Melanie Klein over the level of sophistication and complexity of mental development in infancy. His words, however, are just as applicable to the differences between Daniel Stern (1985) and other contemporary theoreticians of infancy who are disagreeing on the same issue today.

Some of the earliest conceptualizations of infancy, such as those of Sigmund Freud (1911) and Ferenczi (1913), do not seem very plausible from the standpoint of current knowledge. Freud's belief that the infant was hidden behind a "stimulus barrier"—the notion that the senses of sight and hearing did not operate for the first several weeks of life in order to keep the child from being overwhelmed by incoming stimuli—was not confirmed by observation, but nevertheless continued to influence generations of theoreticians who followed. Ferenczi's ideas were even more fanciful. Expanding on Freud, he described the period in the womb as a time when the fetus, if only unconsciously, felt that he or she had everything desirable; and that the time after birth was one of magical hallucinatory omnipotence, when the newborn tried to recapture the perfection of the womb. His formulation continued through additional stages until speech in the child replaced thought and physical movements as a means of representing wishes.

Although these specific hypotheses of Freud and Ferenczi have little credibility today, they do contain concepts which remain central to our understanding of development. These include the importance of the body as a stimulus to mental development and the movement from simple to more complex mental functions and structures as development proceeds from stage to stage.

THE EMERGENCE OF SELF AND OTHER: THE THEORIES OF SPITZ AND MAHLER

The research on infancy has multiplied tenfold in the last decade and can be overwhelming to the beginning student of development. With this thought in mind, I have decided to focus primarily on the work of René Spitz and Margaret Mahler, both clinicians themselves, whose theories of early development are readily conceptualized and compared, thus forming a grid on which to build a more comprehensive picture of the first years of life (see Table 2). Since their ideas extend beyond infancy, the discussion of them will be continued in Chapter Four on the Anal Phase.

We will begin with a consideration of Spitz's theory because his work preceded and influenced Mahler's. Spitz used the term *psychic organizer* to explain the importance of the smile response, the eighth-month anxiety, and negativism. He borrowed the term from embryology where it is used to describe a set of agents and regulating elements which influence subsequent change. Before the emergence of the organizer, for

Table 2. The Theories of Mahler and Spitz

Mahler Separation–individuation theory	Spitz Psychic organizers
1. The autistic phase (0–3 months)	1. The smile response (by 3 months)
2. The symbiotic phase (3–12 months)	2. Stranger anxiety (8 months)
3. The separation–individuation subphase (1–3 years)	3. Negativism (18 months)
4. Object constancy (age 3)	

example, transplanted cells will assume the form and function of the tissue into which they are placed. After the emergence of the organizer they will retain the form and function of the tissue from which they came.

In an analogous way, the smile response, stranger anxiety, and negativism are *indicators* that a new form of psychic organization and complexity has occurred which cannot be reversed. "If the child successfully establishes and consolidates an organizer at the appropriate level, his development can proceed in the direction of the next organizer" (Spitz, 1965, p. 119).

The Smile Response

Spitz described the *smile response* as the first active, directed, intentional behavior; indicating a transition from passivity to activity. Through his research, which is described in detail in *The First Year of Life* (1965), Spitz learned that the infant is responding to a gestalt of the forehead, eyes, and nose, seen straight on and in motion. Since a cardboard "face" will illicit the smile response, the infant is not yet responding to a true object, that is, exclusively to another human being.

Theoretically, the appearance of the smile in response to the gestalt of the human face indicates that a number of profoundly important mental processes are beginning to form. They include the differentiation of internal from external stimuli, reality from fantasy, past from present, and conscious from unconscious.

Since parents almost always remember when their child first smiled, inquiring about the appearance of the first psychic organizer while taking the developmental history is an excellent way to assess the progress of early mental development. Under normal circumstances, the first smile appears between 4 and 6 weeks of age, always by 3 months of age. The absence of the smile by 3 months of age is indicative of profound organic and/or environmental pathology; the causative factors usually already determined from other data. Thus, knowledge of when the smile first occurred is helpful in formulating an impression of early normal development, not pathology.

Stranger Anxiety

Spitz called the second psychic organizer the *eighth-month anxiety*, or as it is more commonly known, *stranger anxiety*. By the middle of the first year (not precisely at 8 months) many children become acutely apprehensive in the presence of a stranger and respond by turning away or crying.

The appearance of stranger anxiety signifies major intrapsychic progression—the infant has developed the capacity to distinguish one human being from another and to recognize the importance of a specific person for his or her well-being. Spitz understood the importance of this progression, stating that the child had now developed the ability to form relationships. He called it the establishment of the true *libidinal object.* Today we would speak of the beginning of *object (people) relationships.*

However, the well-intentioned friends and relatives who do not understand the mental state of the child approach the infant with the expectation that their affection will be immediately returned. When it is not, they assume that the infant does not like them. Parents may become embarrassed or disturbed, apologizing to the guest inappropriately.

Questions about stranger anxiety should be a part of every developmental history. Like the smile response, a confirmation of its presence is an indication that early development was progressing normally. However, not all healthy infants have significant stranger anxiety, and some parents will not remember if it occurred. Consequently, a negative response is not very significant. As with all information gathered during the diagnostic evaluation, the presence or absence of any single finding must be understood in context, in relationship to other relevant data.

The Autistic and Symbiotic
Substages of Separation–Individuation

With this introduction to Spitz's major concepts about the first year of life in place, let us now turn our attention to Mahler's first two subphases. For a more extensive exposition of Mahler's theory, please refer to *The Psychological Birth of the Human Infant* (Mahler, Pine, & Bergman, 1975). Mahler described the first 3 months of life as the *normal autistic stage,* later altering the name to the *pseudoautistic stage.* Both terms are attempts to describe the relatively undeveloped state of higher mental functions at the time of birth and shortly thereafter. The relationship between the infant and the mother (or mothering person) is the key to normal developmental progression because the infant is dependent upon the mother not only for survival, but also for physical and emotional stimulation and for relief from states of intolerable instinctual or environmental stimulation. Mahler (1958) referred to the mother's role as the *external executive ego.*

The second substage, which spans the months from 3 to 12, is called the *normal symbiotic stage.* Attempting to describe how the infantile mind perceives the world and itself, Mahler (1967) hypothesized the gradual awareness of a "need-satisfying object." As the infant becomes more aware of the person (or persons) who respond to his or her smiles and cries, who relieves hunger and other instinctual and environmental pressures, he or she behaves as though infant and mother were an "omnipotent system," a dual entity within a common boundary or membrane.

The critical factor in normal symbiosis is the ability of both infant and mother to send out and receive each other's signals. The infant needs a strong symbiotic involvement with the mother in order to develop a solid sense of self and other, and in order to eventually separate from the mother and to individuate. This principle of intensive engagement of a developmental task at a phase-appropriate time (leading to some degree of mastery) and then gradual disengagement and movement toward the next task (of greater complexity) is applicable to normal development at all points in the life cycle.

The relationship between infant and mother is by no means one-sided because the mother is continually stimulated by the infant who arouses powerful physical sensations (if she is breast-feeding) and emotions. This intensity increases and the scope of such interactions broadens as the child grows, offering both parents the opportunity to rework aspects of their own development, stage by stage, in concert with their offspring.

To summarize normal symbiosis: The distinction between the inner world and external reality is gradually emerging from repeated contact with the mother, particularly through the mother's face, hands, and breast (or bottle) in the context of feeding. The infant behaves as though he or she and mother were an omnipotent system, a dual entity within one common boundary. Self and other are not yet recognized as distinct and separate.

FEEDING AND WEANING

The Role of Frustration and Gratification

Feeding is recognized by most observers of infancy as one of the most important early interactions which stimulate and organize development. Spitz called the oral cavity the *cradle of perception*. Both he and Mahler suggested that the beginning differentiation of self and other, as well as the basic attitude toward life, originated in early feeding experiences. One inborn capacity which is highly developed at birth is the *sucking reflex*. Through its function the infant takes in nourishment and begins to organize experience. For instance, visual perception begins during feeding as the infant gazes at the mother's face while nursing. When the mother promptly relieves hunger pains and responds emotionally and tactily, feeding becomes the basis for relatedness; and the world and those in it are experienced in a positive light.

The emotional interaction between mother and infant, particularly around feeding, was described by Spitz as the *affective climate*. Largely unconscious, this constant, cumulative affective interaction stimulates the emergence of psychic functions.

When the infant does not receive a steady stream of stimulation during the first year of life, the consequences are devastating. Spitz (1945, 1946) studied infants in foundling homes who were nourished but left alone for long periods, thus deprived of the physical and emotional stimulation provided by the mothering person. The infants demonstrated profound developmental delays in all areas and many died by a year of age. Spitz called this syndrome *hospitalism.*

Breast versus Bottle Feeding

According to Anna Freud (1946) eating should be as nonconflictual as possible because of the central role feeding plays in prompting normal emotional development. Satisfaction of hunger is the first experience of instinctual gratification in a child's life. Because the instinctual needs of the infant are of overwhelming urgency and no organized ego exists to delay and control impulses, mother limits the degree of pain and frustration that the infant experiences by *feeding on demand.* But no matter how rapidly she responds to the infant's hunger she will also be associated with the inevitable frustration that the child experiences while waiting for the breast or the bottle.

Consequently, it is not the presence or absence of frustration, but the *pattern* of either rapid response leading to gratification or repeated delay producing prolonged frustration which determines the effect on development. A well-fed baby is a happy baby because he or she begins to develop a sense that life (as represented by the caretakers, primarily through the feeding process) is predictable, safe, and gratifying. This is what Erikson (1963) meant by *basic trust,* which he also related to the early feeding process.

Breast-feeding is nature's way of promoting normal growth and development but bottle-feeding can produce the same result if it is sensitively done. Breast milk is nutritious, warm, and instantly ready. Breast-feeding ensures the mother's participation and provides her with a necessary form of physical gratification as her breasts are emptied. As already described in the discussion of the smile response, the gestalt of the human face, from the distance and position of the infant sucking at the breast, is a powerful psychic organizer. In an atmosphere of mutual gratification of instincts and physical pleasure, the affective interchange between mother and infant is more likely to be positive, enhancing the loving bond between the two.

All these essential, positive aspects of breast-feeding can be approximated in bottle-feeding if their importance is understood by a loving parent. But the possibility of neglect of the infant's physical and emotional needs is greatly increased, for example, by propping up the bottle and thus removing the emotional aspects of the interaction.

This example of how to interact with the child—how theory is translated into practice—is one of many which will be found throughout this book, and illustrates why a knowledge of normal development is so valuable to the clinician both in regard to understanding and treating patients and living life.

Thumb-Sucking

Thumb-sucking is a normal expression of oral pleasure which has been observed *in utero* and may continue throughout the first several years of life. As early mental development proceeds, thumb-sucking becomes increasingly associated with gratification, comfort, and closeness to mother, substituting for her in her absence. As the child moves through the anal and Oedipal phases, the fantasies associated with thumb-sucking change, reflecting the major developmental preoccupations of the moment, such as stresses related to toilet training or Oedipal fears and phobias. Pacifiers, substitute thumbs supplied by the environment, serve the same psychological function.

Weaning

Weaning is the first organized exercise of planned frustration which takes place when the child is old enough to understand what is being taken from him or her, and capable of concentrated verbal and motoric resistance. Weaning is important developmentally because it pushes the child toward the next set of developmental tasks by replacing sucking as the major mechanism for obtaining nourishment; diminishes mother's involvement in the feeding, thus stimulating the separation–individuation process; encourages the gradual repression of oral wishes; and facilitates, through identification with the parents, the ability of the infant to tolerate frustration and control impulses.

Nature promotes weaning toward the end of the first year of life through a combination of infant growth and development, particularly the appearance of teeth and biting, and the return of the menstrual cycle.

Following this lead, weaning from the bottle should be actively initiated by the parents at about 1 year of age and be accomplished gradually over a period of several months. The least important bottle to the child is withdrawn first, followed several weeks later by the second favorite one, and so on, until the child is completely weaned.

Pacifiers may be removed in a similar fashion. Thumb-sucking presents a different problem, however, since the instrument of gratification, the appendage, cannot be taken away. Many children will give up thumb-sucking on their own during the second and third year of life because of their desires to grow up and please the parents. But it may persist beyond this time during such regressive periods as bedtime, separations from parents, and illness. If thumb-sucking continues to be a consistent method of gratification beyond age 3 or 4, a combination of consistent verbalization and encouragement should be used to help the child stop.

THE PREOEDIPAL MOTHER AND FATHER

The Role of Activity versus Passivity

Anna Freud (1946) said that infants have three basic needs: food, oxygen, and *not to be left alone*. The third need underscores the importance of what Spitz called the *mother–child dyad*. Whereas most animals are instinctively capable of caring for themselves at birth, the human being is not. The mother, the human substitute for the instincts, compensates for the immaturity of the central nervous system and the mind, and through her psychological rapport with the infant, compliments the undifferentiated ego, sustaining life and stimulating development.

Another way to characterize early development and describe the infant's emerging picture of the mother–child dyad was suggested by Ruth Mack Brunswick (1940). She described activity versus passivity as the first major antithesis of childhood. The newborn infant is passive and helpless, but almost from the moment of birth onward becomes more active and assertive.

The infant's activity is based, in part, on what the mother does to him or her; however, every act of successful identification with the active mother renders her less necessary. Gradually, the child comes to resent the mother's unavoidable interference with his or her burgeoning activity—for example, the 6-month-old's insistence on holding the bottle and the 12-month-old's refusal to be carried, demanding to walk instead. This anger, toward a loved and feared person, is one of the first experiences of true aggression. Parental response to the activity and aggression (which should be accepting and accommodating) will have a powerful influence on the child's emerging attitudes toward a range of emotions from curiosity to ambition.

Like Spitz and Mahler, Brunswick saw the relationship between mother and child as extraordinarily important. In an attempt to characterize how the infant and toddler must conceptualize the primary caregiver, she defined the term *preoedipal mother*. This is the parent of the first 3 years of life, the mother of the oral and anal phases of development, who is all knowing and all powerful. A figure of overwhelming influence on physical and psychological development, she becomes recognized as the source of all gratification and frustration. In an oversimplified way, we may say that early development is characterized by the child's attempts to separate and individuate from the preoedipal mother, and in the process to assume some of her ability to control and regulate all aspects of life.

Fathers and Infants

Although much of the focus throughout the decades has been on the interaction between infants and mothers, in recent years a great deal of knowledge has been acquired about the relationship between infants and their fathers. The relative neglect of the father's role in infant development in the past was due to the lack of differentiation between maternal and paternal functions in the first year of life—the distinctions and elaboration of differing and interlocking roles will become quite pronounced by the time we consider the Oedipal years—and the need to explore the profoundly influential and still only partially understood infant–mother interaction.

Fathers play particularly important roles in self-object and sexual differentiation, the awareness of physical sensations and knowledge of body parts and actions (Yogmah, 1982), and in the modulation of aggression (Hertzog, 1984). Self-object and sexual differentiation are greatly facilitated by the father's consistent presence and involvement in the infant's care. During the first year of life, the father is increasingly internalized as an important object in his own right and also provides an alternative to the intense symbiotic closeness with the mother. His masculine approach to the infant contrasts with the mother's feminine role and lays the foundation for the beginning differentiation of male from female. A growing awareness of physical sensations and knowledge of body parts is stimulated by the father's tendency to handle the infant's body in a "rougher" fashion than the mother, particularly during play which frequently includes involving the infant's extremities in simulated walking and stretching motions and rapidly moving the infant's entire body through space by rocking or tossing. The modulation of aggression is related to paternal involvement in limit setting and the stimulation of goal-related activities.

For a further consideration of the role of the father in development throughout the life cycle, the reader is referred to *Father and Child: Development and Clinical Perspectives*, edited by Cath, Gurwitt, and Ross (1982) and *Fathers and Their Families*, edited by Cath, Gurwitt, and Gunsberg (1989).

SEXUAL AND COGNITIVE DEVELOPMENT

Up to this point, the ideas presented have focused primarily on the relationship between mother and child and the effect of their interaction on the emergence of basic trust, relationship to self and others, and instinctual gratification and frustration. Now let us turn our attention to the beginnings of sexual and intellectual development. By using Anna Freud's (1965) concept of developmental lines, we may trace a particular theme from phase to phase throughout childhood, indeed, throughout life. I will use this technique repeatedly as we follow the elaboration of basic aspects of human experience.

Core Gender Identity

Sexual awareness in the first year of life is not very evident to the observer, yet the infant is developing what Robert Stoller (1968) called *core gender identity*—the basic, primitive sense of oneself as male or female which is the foundation on which later sexual attitudes and understanding are built.

According to Stoller, this is a complex phenomenon which results from a confluence of biological, environmental, and psychological factors and attitudes. Most likely the process begins *in utero*, stimulated by the admixture of male and female hormones which influence the development of the body and the brain and determine the appearance of the external genitalia. When the external genitalia are clearly of one sex or the other, the child is declared to be a boy or girl, and powerful conscious and unconscious forces are set in motion in the primary caretakers, which cause them to continually bombard the infant with the message, you are a boy, or you are a girl. Under normal circumstances this process continues into the second year of life, resulting by 18 months, in a deeply ingrained, unalterable sense of maleness or femaleness. We will continue to discuss the developmental line of sexual identity formation in each of the developmental phases to follow.

Cognitive Development

Like Sigmund Freud, Piaget used the study of a small number of individuals to formulate a general theory. Although these two giants of twentieth-century thought differed in their area of emphasis, Freud on emotional development, Piaget on intellectual development, both of their theories are developmentally organized and subdivided into stages.

Piaget (1936, 1969) studied the mental processes which allow children to adapt to the environment. He postulated that as information is assimilated, it is organized into categories contained within psychic structures called *schema*. The encounter with new stimuli causes disequilibrium by necessitating the alteration of existing schema and the creation of new ones. Over time, these changes may be organized into stages which are similar in their conceptualization to Freud's. Like the oral and anal phase, for example, Piaget's stages are organized around phase-specific themes and tasks which, when mastered, lead to the acquisition of new mental capacities which then serve as the basis for developmental challenges at the next progressive level (see Table 3).

During the first year of life (and the second), the child is in what Piaget called the *sensorimotor phase*. As conceptualized by Piaget—and, again, it must be remembered that we have no way of confirming what goes on in the infantile mind during this preverbal period—thinking is related to what the child observes in the immediate environment, what is done to him or her by caretakers, and what he or she does to objects with the rudimentary motor skills which develop as the first year progresses. Once again the mother and other primary caretakers are understood to be important stimulants of the developmental process. As was previously noted about sexual development, the developmental line of cognitive development will be traced throughout the life cycle and commented on in other chapters.

Table 3. Piaget's Theory of Cognitive Development

Sensorimotor intelligence	0–18 months
Concrete operations	18 months–12 years
Preoperational period	18 months–7 years
Period of concrete operations	7–12 years
Formal operations	Adolescence and beyond

SELF PSYCHOLOGY AND
THE DEVELOPMENT OF THE SELF

Heinz Kohut

Heinz Kohut (1971, 1977) is the founder of a school of psychological thought called *Self Psychology*. A psychoanalyst, he felt that classical theory was lacking in some areas and incorrect in others, and as a result formulated his own theory, evolving a new set of terms and concepts in the process. Kohut did not elaborate a complete developmental theory, but he did have opinions about the nature of the developmental process.

The key to normal development is the interaction between the child and his or her primary caretakers, in Kohutian terminology, the *selfobjects*. Selfobjects are those primary caretakers who interact with the child in such a positive manner that the child is able to use these interactions to form a clearly defined, comfortable sense of self that is called a *cohesive self-structure* (Wolf, 1988). This structure begins to develop in the infant's mind as a result of repeated experiences with the caregiver who facilitates the emergence of the infant's grandiosity and exhibitionism and accepts these feelings and actions in an *empathetic* (a key concept for Kohut) manner. Over time, as the infant comes to recognize the positive nature of the mirroring selfobject, he or she wishes to merge with the caregiver. (Notice the similarity between these ideas and Mahler's description of the mother–child dyad during the symbiotic subphase.)

Children who manifest signs of healthy development beyond infancy do so because of repeated experiences of empathetic acceptance from important selfobjects throughout childhood, and indeed throughout adolescence and adult life. Pathologic development stems from repeated experiences of less than optimal frustration. When this occurs, the self becomes endangered or fragmented and sexual impulses are expressed in inappropriate ways. Perverse sexuality in adolescence and adulthood results from repeated experiences of selfobject failures.

In contrast to classical analytic theory which postulates the existence of the dual drives, libido and aggression, Kohut considered sexual and aggressive impulses to be aspects of the healthy self. As previously described, the ability to love self and others stems from empathetic interactions with selfobjects. The same is true in regard to aggression (Moore & Fine, 1990, pp. 174–176). Normal aggression, which has a range of expression from assertiveness to competitiveness, emerges from repeated experience with optimal amounts of frustration. Gradually, the child learns to do for himself or herself, mirroring the controlled aggression central to parental limit setting. When anger is stimulated by experiences of less than optimum frustration, it is directed toward others with an intent to harm. Inherent in this notion, as in classical psychoanalytic theory, is the belief that all children experience both kinds of encounters with self-objects—the long-range effect determined by which of the two is most frequent. Narcissistic rage which results from the chronic failures in empathy is expressed as cruelty, hatred, and the desire to attack others, in contrast to normal aggression which is channeled into assertiveness and goal-directed behavior.

Kohut's views on Oedipal development differ from those of classical psychoanalysis (see Chapter Five). He considers the Oedipal complex to be a pathologic construction, resulting from unempathetic selfobject responses during the Oedipal years, such as overly stimulating or punitive reactions to the child's sexuality and aggression. By contrast, the term *Oedipal stage* is used to describe normative experience during the Oedipal years, characterized by acceptance of the child's sexuality and competitiveness without a pattern of punitiveness or seductive response by the parental selfobjects.

As the child moves through subsequent developmental stages, if the interactions with the selfobject are characterized by a predominance of positive interactions and a minimum of empathic failures, the nuclear self of the child will crystallize and gradually replace the primary caregiver(s) in importance.

Empathy is emphasized as a therapeutic tool by self psychology. It refers to therapeutic immersion in the subjective world of the patient in order to gain understanding and insight which can be communicated to the patient at an appropriate time. Once the therapist gains a detailed understanding of the patient through empathy, he or she is ready to facilitate the phenomenon of *transmuting internalization*. As the therapist frustrates the patient in optimal, nontraumatic ways, unlike the experiences with familial selfobjects which were instrumental in producing the disorder of the self which brought the patient for treatment, he or she gradually learns to perform vital selfobject functions in the absence of involvement with the selfobject of the therapist, thus producing a healthy transformation of the self.

Those readers who wish to learn more about Kohut's ideas should read *The Analysis of the Self: A Systematic Approach to the Psychoanalytic Treatment of Narcissistic Personality Disorders* (1971) and *Restoration of the Self* (1977). Critical reviews have been written by Wallerstein (1981) and Rangell (1982). An elaborate presentation of the development of a sense of self may be found in Chapter Seven of *Psychoanalytic Theories of Development* (1990) by Phyllis and Robert Tyson.

The Self in Infancy—Daniel Stern

Operating primarily but not exclusively within a self-psychology framework, Daniel Stern, a prominent infant researcher, has evolved his own theory of the emergence of the self in infancy. Putting aside much of psychoanalytic theory, but retaining the emphasis on the mother–child interaction, Stern (1974) used his detailed observations of infants and their mothers to formulate his theory. Seeing the infant as exquisitely attuned to respond to his or her mother's caregiving from birth onward, Stern described four different senses of self which emerge during infancy. They are the *emergent self* (0–2 months), the *core self* (2–6 months), the *subjective self* (7–9 months), and the *verbal self* (9 months into the second year). Stern's ideas will be presented here, but not the fascinating research methods and data on which they are based. For a more detailed consideration, the reader is referred to his *The Interpersonal World of the Infant* (1985).

Stern describes the sense of an emergent self during the first 2 months of life. The newborn is occupying "some kind of presocial, precognitive, preorganized life phase" (1985, p. 37). In addition to being interested in what the infant's sense of self is, Stern also wonders how the infant experiences the social world. As a result of the revolution in infant research during the past 20 years which has greatly increased our ability to observe and study this early, preverbal period of life, Stern feels that there are enough data to conclude that there exists an organization in the process of formation, "a sense of self that will remain active for the rest of life" (p. 38).

At 2 to 3 months of age, a critical transformation occurs in the infant which Stern called the *core self*. At this time infants begin to approach others with an "organized perspective" (p. 69) which gives observers the impression that there exists

> an integrated sense of themselves as distinct and coherent bodies, with control over their own actions, ownership of their own affinity, a sense of continuity, and a sense of other people as distinct and separate interactants. (p. 69)

Stern was openly critical of developmental theory, particularly that of Mahler, which does not describe the infant at this age as possessing an integrated sense of self. He suggested that recent research disproves the belief that "infants go through an extended period of self/other undifferentiation and that only very slowly, sometime toward the end of the first year of life, do they differentiate a sense of self and other" (p. 69). In its place is the notion that the first order of business for the infant is creating an interpersonal world; creating a sense of "core self" and "core other" (p. 70) which is established between 2 and 7 months of age.

The next quantum leap forward in the evolution of the self occurs between 7 and 9 months, at the same time as Spitz's stranger anxiety and Mahler's symbiotic phase. Then the "infant discovers that he or she has a mind and that other people have minds as well" (p. 124). Stern called this the sense of a *subjective self*. At this point awareness is simple—"I want a cookie" or "this is exciting" (p. 124)—and includes the idea that the infant's subjective experience is similar to and can be shared with others. The emergence of the subjective self catapults the infant into a new "domain of intersubjective relatedness" (p. 125) which transforms the nature of his or her relationship to others and vice versa.

Toward the middle of the second year of life children begin to represent things in their minds through the use of signs and symbols. The emergence of these functions makes language and symbolic play possible. Stern called this period of time, which coincides with the second half of Piaget's sensorimotor period, *the sense of a verbal self*. With the acquisition of language "the self and the other have different and distinct personal world knowledge as well as a new medium of exchange with which to create shared meaning" (p. 162).

The emergence of language greatly expands the capacity for relatedness but also "drives a wedge" between two simultaneous forms of interpersonal experience: "as it is lived and as it is verbally represented" (p. 162). Because experience in the domains of emergent, core, and interpersonal relatedness—which continues irrespective of the development of language and is not replaced or subsumed by the sense of verbal self—can be expressed only partially through words, the emergence of language can cause a split in the experience of the self. This split is fundamental to the formation of neurotic behavior later in life. "Language forces a space between interpersonal experience as lived and as represented. And it is exactly across this space that the connections and associations that constitute neurotic behavior may form" (p. 182).

Stern's ideas have stimulated a productive ferment in psychodynamic thinking and theory building. By insisting that the infant is infinitely more complex and organized at a mental level than suggested by Spitz, Mahler, and others, he questions the usefulness of their theories and raises the more basic issue of what it is possible to know about the nature of the human mind before the appearance of language. His critics contend that Stern infers a level of mental sophistication which does not exist and can only be inferred. Another area of controversy involves the clinical applicability of these ideas; more specific is the infantile self identifiable in the treatment of older children and adults, and if so how is it represented? For a thorough discussion of these complex issues, the reader is referred to Monograph Five of the American Psychoanalytic Association, *The Significance of Infant Observational Research for Clinical Work with Children, Adolescents, and Adults* (1989), edited by Dowling and Rothstein.

EVIDENCE OF ORALITY IN LATER DEVELOPMENT

The internalized residue from the engagement of phase-specific developmental tasks continues to exert an influence on normality and pathology in all subsequent phases. For example, the importance of food and oral gratification as organizers of social and emotional experience may be traced throughout childhood and adulthood.

During the anal phase, such basic oral themes and experiences as the direct relationship between mother and food, weaning, and thumb-sucking are still in evidence. But as the child continues to individuate and becomes more active, he or she exerts a much greater degree of control over these processes and interactions. Anal preoccupations and issues begin to influence how the child reacts to food and feeding. Many times the toddler refuses to be fed, clamping the jaw shut or turning the head, insisting instead on feeding himself or herself with an inevitable degree of messiness. Strong food preferences begin to appear, associated with the color, texture, taste, and temperature. Unless the parent is respectful and accepting of these behaviors, eating may become a source of significant conflict and pathology.

During the Oedipal phase sexuality is understood by the child in oral and anal terms. For example, mother gets pregnant by swallowing something. The baby grows in the "tummy" and comes out through the belly button or anus.

In latency, buying certain food products becomes associated with emerging concepts of masculinity or femininity; for example, eating Wheaties in order to become a football or baseball star. Oral regression remains readily identifiable; for example, having "a pain in the tummy for Mommy" in association with the experience of going away to camp for the first time.

In adolescence, food fads, inconsistent attitudes toward eating, and rejection of favorite family dishes are all aspects of the major physical and psychological changes which characterize the tumultuous transition from childhood to adulthood. Pathologic conditions, such as anorexia nervosa, illuminate the interplay among oral drives, infantile sexual themes, and separation and individuation themes.

In adulthood, eating, a major source of pleasure and social interaction, becomes increasingly associated with the maintenance of health and body integrity. Oral pathology is evident in obesity and addictions to nicotine, drugs, and alcohol. Concepts about orality have also been used to describe aspects of character development; for instance, the demanding, whining, insatiable behavior of the "oral character."

Although this may appear to be an oversimplication, there is much clinical validity to the concept that degrees of pathology are related to stages of development in early childhood. This idea grew out of the recognition that individuals with severe pathological conditions, such as borderline states, narcissistic personalities, and even some psychoses, often experienced severe disruptions in development during the preoedipal years of life. By contrast, those individuals with less severe pathology (neurotics, for example) usually had relatively normal developmental experiences during the first three years of life but were unable to master Oedipal themes. Psychodynamic theories of various pathologic states are based on these equations:

Preoedipal disruption = Severe forms of pathology

Unresolved Oedipal conflict =
Neuroses and less severe forms of pathology

CHAPTER 4

The Anal Phase (Ages 1–3)

The years between 1 and 3 are a time of explosive physical growth and psychological development. During this relatively brief period of time, toddlers develop a strong sense of self and the ability to maintain relationships with others; the capacity to walk and talk; and the ability to utilize and control the body, mind, and environment in sophisticated ways. The "terrible twos" are real enough, but only for the parents; for the child, they are a time of wonderment and excitement as horizons broaden and the world becomes the subject of exploration and amusement.

In this phase of development, as in the oral phase, theoreticians continue to assign enormous importance to the role of the mother. This assignment will disturb some readers because it seems to suggest that no one other than the mother can play a role in promoting healthy infant and toddler development. This is not so, and for this reason I will use a number of different terms, such as *mother, mothering person, caretakers,* and *primary caregivers,* to describe those individuals who care for very young children. However, it is important to recognize that no one is as equipped to promote normal development as the two biological parents who love each other and their offspring. Furthermore, because infants require the physical and psychological interactions which we associate with the terms *mother* and *father,* all other caretakers approximate these functions to the best of their ability.

THE EMERGENCE OF SELF AND OTHER: THE THEORIES OF SPITZ AND MAHLER

With this brief introduction behind us let us begin our discussion of the anal phase, as we did the oral phase, with a consideration of the ideas of Spitz and Mahler.

The Third Psychic Organizer, "No"

Spitz placed great emphasis on the importance of locomotion as a stimulus to psychological development, particularly on object–people relationships. Once the toddler begins to walk, at approximately 1 year of age, the basic nature of his or her relationship with the world changes. During infancy, the interaction between mother and child was organized by tactile and visual contact, particularly in the context of feeding; now their relationship is increasingly shaped by the toddler's ability to create a physical distance between them. As he or she begins to venture away, verbal communication becomes a necessary part of their relationship. In fact, Spitz hypothesized that in the course of human evolution walking was a major stimulus to the development of language.

This newfound ability of the toddler to walk, climb, and explore forces mother and father (and other primary caretakers) to repeatedly curb the child's initiative out of a concern for his or her safety. Increasingly they must say "no," shaking their heads from side to side.

These prohibitions cause frustration which the healthy toddler does not readily tolerate. Caught in a conflict between his or her need for physical and emotional closeness and the drive for autonomy and independence, the toddler solves the dilemma by developing the defense mechanism of *identification with the aggressor*. By using the disciplinarian's word and gesture, the child remains identified with the caregiver and, as Anna Freud put it, is still free to attack the outside world. Once this mechanism is established, the stubbornness of the second year begins in earnest. Spitz's third psychic organizer is now in place. Erikson (1963) described the toddler's dilemma at this point in the life cycle as *autonomy versus shame and doubt*. Muscular maturation pushes the toddler to experiment with two simultaneous sets of social modalities, holding on and letting go. Because the toddler has little ability to discriminate or control these new expressions of assertion and aggression, the environment must support him or her with a benevolent firmness. If this does not occur, the toddler is in danger, "for if denied the gradual and well-guided experience of the autonomy of free choice (or, if indeed weakened by an initial loss of trust) the child will turn against himself all his urge to discriminate and to manipulate. He will over-manipulate himself, he will develop a precocious conscience" (Erikson, 1963, p. 252). The result will be the emergence of shame and doubt, emotions which smother the child's drive for autonomy and undermine future development.

The Separation–Individuation Subphase

The first two subphases of Mahler's separation–individuation theory, the autistic and symbiotic, occur during the first year of life. The third and last subphase, also confusingly called separation–individuation, covers the period from 12 to 36 months and leads to the attainment of object constancy.

Like Spitz, Mahler, Pine, and Bergman (1975) viewed locomotion as a great catalyzing influence on the development of the ego. As walking exposes the infant to deliberate bodily separation from the mother, psychological separation and individuation must inevitably follow. Indeed, psychological separation from the symbiotic common membrane with mother is as inevitable as biological birth. Only a fair degree of emotional acceptance and "communicative matching" on mother's part is necessary for this to occur. When parental acceptance is present, the toddler is at the "peak of elation," free to explore the world while still sharing in mother's magical powers.

Mahler considered the toddler's negativism to be a healthy expression of the drive toward autonomy. But the negativism results in emotional as well as physical distance and precipitates various forms of regression (which we will consider under the heading Developmental Disturbances of the Toddler). At this time of vulnerable self-esteem, the toddler needs mother's consistent presence and the support of father and other caregivers in order to control the regressive fear/wish for reengulfment by the mother, which is expressed in the characteristic fear of this phase, *separation anxiety.*

The Rapprochement Crisis

The aspect of Mahler's (1963) theory during the second year of life which has greatest clinical relevance is the *rapprochement crisis.* This normal interaction, initiated by the toddler between 14 and 24 months, consists of repeated attempts to return to mother and involve her in play, exploration, and the acquisition of newly acquired skills. When mother is available and actively participates with encouragement and enthusiasm, the toddler is emotionally refueled and ready to venture again, alone, into the ever expanding world. But even under the best of circumstances both mother and child experience intervals of ambivalence and frustration as they repeatedly work through the intense feelings of reunion and separation.

The term *rapprochement crisis* has both normative and pathological connotations. In the normative sense, the word *crisis* conveys both the turmoil and intensity in the interaction and the importance which Mahler attached to rapprochement. In the pathological sense, crisis refers to the toddler's responses when mother is unavailable or does not respond—

active-pursuit behavior followed by temper tantrums, clinging, whining, and sleep disturbances.

Object Constancy

At approximately age 3, the separation–individuation process culminates in the emergence of a capacity which is at the core of all human interaction for the remainder of life. *Object constancy* may be defined as the capacity to maintain mental representations of mother and other important persons for extended periods of time in their absence. So equipped, the young child is capable of providing himself or herself with emotional sustenance and relatedness. Those who provide definition and meaning to life are captured intrapsychically where they can be related to and manipulated through fantasy. The engagement and resolution of the Oedipal complex would be impossible without object constancy, another example of how capacities acquired at one phase of development become the basis for engagement of new, more complicated tasks at the next phase.

In the preschool years, the ability to maintain object constancy is jeopardized by prolonged absences from the primary caretakers. As childhood progresses, this danger diminishes. In adults, the ability to maintain mental representations of figures from the past even after prolonged absence is almost unlimited. For example, think of a special childhood friend or college roommate whom you have not seen for many years. The mental image of the person can be readily recalled along with associated memories and feelings. Meeting such an individual after an absence of many years demonstrates the tenacity of such images and is often shocking because of the discrepancy between the mental picture of the way he or she was and their appearance and behavior in the present.

Self-constancy is the compliment to object constancy. By the middle of the second year, toddlers begin to think of themselves as separate beings. As the capacity for mental representation increases and the separation–individuation process proceeds, the sense of self grows until a stable core of identity is firmly established. In Kohutian terminology, the emergence of a cohesive self structure (Wolf, 1988) conveys the same idea, that because of consistently positive interactions with his or her selfobjects the toddler is developing an integrated sense of self which is the bedrock on which future healthy development rests.

Applications of Separation–Individuation Theory

Separations. As is abundantly clear from the theories of Spitz and Mahler, infants and toddlers cannot tolerate prolonged separations from their primary caretakers without negative effects. Easy normal development is best promoted by consistent parental presence in a setting in which the child is free to leave the parent and affect a rapprochement when desired. But parents have needs, too, including breaks from the vigorous demands of raising a toddler. Unfortunately, the parents' need to work and play does not always resonate with the toddler's need for continuity. Consequently, the answers which we provide to parental questions about separations are not always the ones they would like to hear.

The following intervals are general guidelines written from the point of view of the optimal promotion of normal development. It should be remembered, however, that children are resilient and thrive in less than ideal circumstances. Furthermore, it is a *pattern* of prolonged absences rather than a single or occasional one which is most likely to be detrimental.

During the first 3 years of life, parental absences should be limited to 1 or 2 days. During the Oedipal phase this interval can be comfortably extended up to a week, depending upon the tolerance of the individual child. Most latency-aged children can manage absences of 1 to 2 weeks without undue anxiety or regression. Normal early adolescents have a well-developed capacity for object constancy and are not vulnerable to parental absences in the sense described for younger children. However, they are in continuous need of the structure, judgment, and limit setting which their parents provide. Consequently, mature caretakers should be provided in the event of parental absence.

Substitute Caretakers. As previously stated, the healthy development of infants and toddlers is most likely to be promoted by the active care of two biological parents who love each other and are invested in raising their child. When the above circumstances do not or cannot exist because of the need to work, divorce, or other realistic considerations, alternative arrangements must be made. In order to approximate the relationship between parents and child, substitute caretakers should be physically and emotionally intact, invested in the child as an individual, and able to remain involved for an extended period of time. If caretaking must occur outside the child's home or in a day-care setting, the same persons should care for the child on a regular basis, and the ratio of adult to child should be as small as possible.

Relationship to Diagnosis and Treatment. Mahler's theory, which grew in part out of her experience as a clinician, has been used as both a diagnostic and treatment tool. Mahler (1952) herself conceptualized childhood psychoses in terms of autistic and symbiotic types. Because the capacity for relating to others is such an integral part of human experience, separation–individuation theory has also been used to define severe, but nonpsychotic forms of pathology, such as the narcissistic and borderline states. The reader who is interested in pursuing this area of study may refer to the works of Kernberg (1975) and Kohut (1977).

The rapprochement crisis is used by some clinicians to explain and interpret transference phenomena. The basic idea involved (Kramer & Akhtar, 1988) is that patients who experienced significant impairments in the rapprochement process during the second year of life will recreate their traumatic experience in the relationship to the therapist. The defects and conflicts related to rapprochement can thus be conceptualized and interpreted by the clinician.

THE TRANSITIONAL OBJECT

Another prominent theoretician who studied the infant's physical and psychological separation from mother was Winnicott (1953). He is responsible for explaining the importance of teddy bears and blankets to infants and toddlers. Using the term *transitional object*, Winnicott suggested that these soft, fuzzy objects begin to have a special significance during the second half of the first year of life because they represent aspects of the infant and toddler's relationship to mother. By choosing and using a transitional object to represent mother, the toddler is able, through fantasy, to remain connected to her during periods of separation. Toddlers may also use transitional phenomena—sounds, words, songs, and other verbal expressions closely associated with mother—for the same purpose.

Transitional objects are used by both sexes in the same manner and frequency, most likely because the processes of separation and individuation are basically the same for boys and girls. However, not all children require a transitional object to successfully negotiate the separation–individuation process. Thus, as with most other data, the clinician must relate information about transitional objects and phenomena to other information before drawing diagnostic conclusions.

Famous and Infamous Blankets

Probably the most famous transitional object in existence is Linus's blanket from the comic strip, *Peanuts*. His intense attachment to the blanket illustrates a frequently encountered problem faced by parents and clinicians—how to help children give them up. Although Linus's blanket may be the most famous one in the world, it is not necessarily the most infamous one. That distinction may belong to the blanket of a patient of mine whom I shall call Shelly. When she was 4 years and 7 months old, I received a frantic call from her mother asking what she should do. Shelly's blanket was "gone"! As I asked questions the following story emerged. The child had been deeply attached to her blanket from the age of 1, refusing to venture anywhere without it. As time passed, the mother found it necessary to occasionally wash the blanket, which had become tattered, dirty, and smelly. On such occasions, Shelly would stand longingly under her transitional object while it hung on the clothesline to dry, tantalizingly out of reach. The immediate crisis was precipitated by the fact that the blanket, reduced by the years of constant use to a rag, had gone into the washing machine—and had not come out!

Shelly survived the loss of her blanket and went on to become a lawyer. But her parents could have saved her and themselves considerable anxiety and distress if they had helped Shelly give up her blanket when it was no longer necessary developmentally. Just as sucking on the breast or bottle does not further the developmental process as the second year of life progresses, neither does strong attachment to a transitional object after object constancy is achieved. Like weaning from the bottle, if the child has not given up the transitional object on his or her own as the fourth year of life progresses, the parents should structure an active weaning process from it. Since the child of 3 or 4 years has the capacity for language, words as well as limits may be employed. After explaining that the child can learn to be comfortable without the transitional object, and therefore feel more grown up, a gradual process of withdrawal is initiated. For example, the treasure may first be restricted to the house, then the bedroom, next to the bed at bedtime, and finally to a drawer or shelf where it remains on a permanent basis, ready to be rediscovered many years later as a remnant of a distant past, the conflict surrounding its surrender forgotten.

DEVELOPMENTAL DISTURBANCES OF THE TODDLER

The *terrible twos* is a commonly used term to describe the behavior of the toddler. We have just considered how some of the "symptoms" observed at this time are related to the stresses involved in the separation–individuation process. Anna Freud (1965) has provided additional insights into this behavior under the title "The Developmental Disturbances of the Toddler."

The manifestations are tied to the height of anal sadism and express its trends in part directly through destructiveness, messiness, and motor restlessness, and in part reactively, through clinging, inability to separate, whining, and chaotic affective states (including temper tantrums). For all its severity and pathological appearance the whole syndrome is short lived. It remains in force while there are no other than motor outlets for the child's drive derivatives and affects, and it disappears or decreases in intensity as soon as new pathways for discharge have been opened up, especially by the acquisition of speech. (A. Freud, 1965, pp. 161–162)

Thus, this is a brief interval in which there is a natural imbalance between the powerful, maturing body, exploding with new potential, and the ability of the mind to contain and channel the newly emergent feelings and functions. As the ego gradually acquires the ability to control the drives, a new, more comfortable equilibrium is established. This will not be the last time that we will encounter such an imbalance between body and mind. In fact, the most outstanding example occurs in adolescence when the physical maturational events surrounding puberty upset the very comfortable equilibrium which existed in the golden age of childhood (late latency) and force the major psychological reorganization of adolescence.

Let us consider the components of the developmental disturbances of the toddler, one by one. The *destructiveness* commonly seen in toddlers is an expression of unbridled aggression and curiosity operating in the absence of the concepts of cause and effect and value. The parental task is to control the aggression without stifling the developing curiosity, since ambition and curiosity are highly valuable aspects of normal learning. *Messiness* is a natural consequence of exploration in the absence of a need for orderliness and organization. *Motor restlessness* stems from the desire to continually practice the new motor skills of walking, running, talking, and eye–hand coordination. Although monotonous for adults, such activities are just as enjoyable to the toddler on the one hundredth repetition as they were on the first.

It follows from this understanding that toddlers should be provided with a safe place in which to explore and practice. Because they do not yet have the ability to recognize danger, they must be protected from cutting themselves on sharp objects, falling down stairs, or swallowing harmful substances. They should not be punished for destructiveness or messiness, nor should they be required to clean up after themselves. Motor restlessness should be contained rather than squashed through the provision of a safe place in which to practice and the structuring of a routine which includes adequate amounts of nutrition, rest, and supervision.

Temper Tantrums

Temper tantrums are the most striking example of the whining, chaotic, affective states described by Anna Freud. Although they are normal occurrences during this phase of development, they are characterized by a genuine loss of control of both feelings and behavior. In the midst of a true temper tantrum, the toddler will usually throw himself or herself on the floor, kicking, screaming, and crying. Because this is a genuinely terrifying experience for the child, the parental goal should be to help the child regain control as soon as possible. This is accomplished by remaining in physical and verbal contact (rather than through isolation and punishment), calmly providing support and reassurance until the tantrum is over. Fake tantrums, used by older children to manipulate and control parental interactions, are readily distinguishable from genuine tantrums and should be treated like any other attempt to test limits, with explanations and consistent firmness. Parents of toddlers frequently ask when it is appropriate to spank a child as a means of discipline. The use of physical punishment as a consistent disciplinary tool is inappropriate at any age, and is usually initiated by the relatively healthy parent as a rationalization for retaliating against the child who has provoked the parent beyond his or her limits. A rare swat across the bottom is not likely to harm either the parent or the child. However, it should be understood that the child's attitude toward aggression in later life, whether directed toward himself or herself or others, is strongly influenced by the pattern of limit setting and discipline to which they were exposed as children. Those children who were managed with kind firmness will treat their children in a similar fashion. Adults who were abused as children are very likely, without therapeutic intervention, to abuse their own children.

Sleep Disturbances

Sleep disturbances occur during this phase of development for the same reasons as the developmental disturbances of the toddler. Gesell and Ilg (1943) saw them as one of the most commonly observed behaviors of the 15- to 30-month-old child. Nagera (1966) suggested that they are almost universal during the anal phase. In fact, although their etiology differs, sleep disturbances are a very common phenomenon during the first three developmental phases, oral, anal, and Oedipal.

Nagera divided sleep disturbances during the anal phase into three types. The first type is related to the immaturity of the ego. During the second year of life, children are still vulnerable to the absence of the mother. Going to sleep means leaving her. In addition, as fears and nightmares begin to appear during the third year of life (precursors of Oedipal stage behavior), the toddler is vulnerable because of the limited ability to distinguish fantasy from reality. The tiger in the closet is real.

The second type of sleep disturbance is related to the emergence of the new capacities previously described. Toddlers do not want to go to sleep and give up the pleasure of practicing. Consequently, bedtime may be difficult for toddler and parent alike. The situation may be managed as follows. A regular bedtime should be established during the first year of life. As the second year progresses, the routine leading up to bedtime may be expanded to include a small snack, a bath, and a few quiet minutes with mom or dad reading from a favorite book, thus shifting the focus from intense motor activity to a peaceful calm. Despite all of this, the moment of truth will arrive when the parent must say good night, turn out the light, and leave the bedroom with screams of protest echoing in his or her ears, if only for a few seconds or minutes. Inevitable requests for a drink of water or another story should be consistently refused. If this pattern is repeated calmly but firmly, day after day, the toddler will internalize the routine. Tolerance of frustration will increase and the external control of impulses will be gradually replaced by an internal one which will serve the toddler well for the remainder of life.

The third type of sleep disturbance is related to anal-phase issues and conflicts. The capacity for internal conflict, the intrapsychic struggle between impulses and self-imposed limitations and restrictions, is beginning to occur for the first time as the child internalizes parental demands and expectations. An excellent example of anal-phase conflict was described by Berta Bornstein (1953) in her treatment of a 2½-year-old girl who was in the midst of toilet training. She was afraid to go to sleep because of the fear of soiling her bed. Behind the fear was an intense conflict over the wish to soil and the fear of losing mother's love.

Attitudes toward Food

Another reflection of the toddler's growing autonomy and complexity is his or her attitude toward food. Whereas infants have a limited diet and do not discriminate between foods, toddlers have strong food preferences. In addition, during the second year of life healthy toddlers insist on controlling the acts of eating and drinking themselves.

Foods are touched and smelled as well as tasted. They are squeezed, crushed, and thrown with the fingers as well as with forks and spoons. Some are preferred or rejected because of color, texture, or temperature as well as taste. Following the dictum presented in Chapter Three that eating should be a nonconflictual pleasure, parents should encourage the joyful exploration of food with all the senses as well as the active manipulation of foodstuffs and the acts of eating and drinking.

Because of their limited frustration tolerance, it is difficult for toddlers to wait when they are hungry. Therefore, some eating should be allowed between parental mealtimes. Once served, toddlers (or older children for that matter) should not be forced to finish their plate or taste all foods presented to them. Nor should neatness or table manners be emphasized. They are beyond the capacity of the toddler and will become, through the desire to identify with the parents' and older siblings' more mature behavior, an integral part of the child's interest and desire during the Oedipal phase and latency.

Parents who are particularly controlling and fastidious may react strongly to the toddler's independence and messiness. This reaction can be minimized to a degree by placing an oilcloth under the high chair and utilizing spillproof cups and nonbreakable dishes and utensils. The attitudes toward eating which are formulated during the first 3 years of life are the basis for a lifetime of healthful, pleasurable nourishment, or the foundation for eating disorders later in life.

TOILET TRAINING

Before beginning a focused discussion of toilet training *per se*, let us consider the biological and environmental factors which are involved and Anna Freud's (1965) developmental line "From Wetting and Soiling to Bowel and Bladder Control."

Biological and Environmental Factors

The biological factors include the increased awareness and control of the lower half of the body, the actions of retaining and expelling urine and feces, and the body products themselves. The environmental influences are centered in the primary caretakers' attitudes toward these actions and products and the process of toilet training.

As myelinization of the lower extremities progresses during the second and third years of life, the toddler develops the capacity to consciously open and close the anal and urethral sphincters. This newfound ability occurs at the same time as the growing awareness of body openings and the products that come from them. Toddlers find the actions and the products highly pleasurable. Consequently urine and feces are to be touched, smelled, tasted, and played with; not reacted to with avoidance and disgust. Thus, there is nothing about the biological factors which pushes the toddler toward toilet training.

That stimulus comes from the parents and is gradually accepted by the toddler. In the midst of the separation–individuation subphase, he or she is increasingly aware of their power and importance. This awareness stimulates a conflict between the pleasures associated with the freedom to wet and soil and the demands of the environment for cleanliness. Eventually, the desire to complete development, to grow up, and the need for parental love and approval override the pleasures associated with the biological factors and the child is trained.

The actions of withholding and expelling urine and feces and the body products themselves become increasingly associated in the toddler's mind with his or her awareness of and feelings about the primary caretakers. As the toddler's attitudes toward his or her body products become increasingly apparent, eventually focusing on the demand that he or she be trained, the actions associated with urinating and defecating and the products themselves become vehicles for expressing a wide range of thoughts and feelings about the parents—love, hate, stubbornness, and compliance to name just a few.

From Wetting and Soiling to Bowel and Bladder Control

Anna Freud (1965) described the developmental line "From Wetting and Soiling to Bowel and Bladder Control" in an attempt to offer a method of toilet training and depict the intrapsychic changes which take place in the child as a result of the prolonged interaction between parent and child. Spanning four developmental phases, the formulation is a superb example of the practical and theoretical usefulness of the developmental framework. The goal of the developmental line is not only to help form the ability to comfortably control the elimination processes, but to stimulate adaptive intrapsychic attitudes and capabilities toward self and others; a far cry from those approaches which propose toilet training in a morning or 24 hours.

This developmental line is divided into four phases. The first, which begins at birth, is described as the complete freedom to wet and soil. It continues until the toilet-training process is initiated. The second phase, active toilet training, should not begin before the child is developmentally ready to participate in the process, at approximately age 2. The reasons for choosing age 2 will be explained shortly.

Anna Freud described the parental attitudes which facilitate the toilet-training process as follows:

> If she succeeds in remaining sensitive to the child's needs and as identified
> with them as she is usually with regard to feeding, she will mediate sympa-
> thetically between the environmental demands for cleanliness and the child's
> opposite anal and urethral tendencies; in that case toilet training will proceed
> gradually, uneventfully and without upheavals. (1965, p. 74)

The interaction between caretakers and child just described is repeated many times over the months and years of active toilet training.
When the process proceeds in a positive fashion, Phase 3—the acceptance
by the child of the environmental demands for controlled urination and
defecation—overlaps Phase 2 and results in far-reaching intrapsychic
changes in the child.

During Phase 3,

> the child accepts and takes over the mother's and the environment's attitudes
> to cleanliness and through identification, makes them an integral part of his
> ego and superego demands; from then onward, the striving for cleanliness is
> an internal, not an external, percept, and inner barriers against urethral and
> anal wishes are set up through the defense activity of the ego, in the well
> known form of repression and reaction formation. (p. 74)

At this point, the child manifests the typical disgust toward urine and
feces found in all older children and adults and demonstrates the increased ability to control powerful feelings, particularly aggression, which
accompany the newfound ability to control the body and its products.

But this is not the end of the story or the developmental line. That
concept is contained in Phase 4, when bowel and bladder control becomes wholly secure, an autonomous ego function disconnected from its
environmental origins. At this point, sometime during latency, bowel and
bladder control lapses do not occur, even at times of stress; and the use
of the toilet is completely disconnected from parental knowledge, dictates, or support. In the physically and psychologically healthy individual, this state continues for the remainder of life or until some point in
old age when physical infirmity undermines the long-standing autonomy
and competence of bowel and bladder function.

The Mechanics of Toilet Training

With these concepts in mind, let us turn our attention to the process of toilet training which may begin at approximately 2 years of age
because by that time the toddler is physically and psychologically capable of complying. In order to cooperate, the child must be able to
understand what the parents want, to consciously control the anal and
urethral sphincters, and to communicate with the caretakers about his or
her intentions.

Toilet training should be an *active* process, initiated by primary care-takers. After the parental expectations have been communicated verbally, all diapers are removed, during the day and at night, and replaced by training pants. The consistent use of training pants rather than diapers (even though it means wet clothes, floors, and beds for a period of time) both represents the parental expectation and focuses the child's attention on the mechanisms of urination and defecation. At the same time, a potty chair is introduced and explained. Its use allows the toddler to sit comfortably with feet planted firmly on the floor, thus eliminating concerns about falling or balancing.

Some children will begin to comply rather quickly while others will resist mightily, sometimes for extended periods of time. In either event, compliance should be responded to with praise; and resistance with the nonpunitive expectation of compliance in the future. If the ideas contained in Anna Freud's developmental line are understood, the adults involved will recognize that their goals of physical compliance and intra-psychic mastery can only be achieved over a period of years.

Under ideal circumstances the toilet-training process will take place in the presence of physical health and environmental stability. Delays or the regressive loss of control can be expected during times of illness and environment instability, such as the birth of a sibling or parental separation. In most instances, consistent control of bowel and bladder functions, day and night, will be achieved between ages 3 to 4 and complete autonomy by ages 7 or 8.

Pathologic outcomes occur when parents fail to actively train the child, usually out of an unconscious fear of their own aggression which is stimulated by the toddler's resistance, or when they are unusually controlling and severe. Enuresis and encopresis may result from either approach. When a consistent expectation is not presented to the toddler, he or she is not helped to develop the ego skills needed to control body products and feelings. Such an approach to toilet training is often observed in association with other inconsistencies in limit-setting interactions, such as weaning and establishing a consistent bedtime. In addition to problems with bowel and bladder control, these children often have difficulty in social relationships with peers and adults and are frequently observed to be self-centered and immature. Severe toilet training has been related to enuresis, encopresis, and withholding of feces, and the obsessive-compulsive neurosis. In these instances, the conflict between parent and child may become internalized, repeatedly expressed through the symptomatic behavior.

SEXUAL AND COGNITIVE DEVELOPMENT

The Awareness of Genital Differences

During the first 18 months of life, the core gender identity, the basic sense of maleness or femaleness, is established. The major element which is added to this undefined sense of gender during the second and third year of life is the awareness of the existence of two different sets of genitals. In the process of this discovery, the boy and the girl further define their own gender identity by developing a more complex understanding of the appearance and workings of their sexual equipment.

As the boy becomes more aware of his penis, urinary stream, and the sensation that comes from the penis during flaccid and erect states, he increasingly wishes to involve the parents in this new and exciting aspect of his life. Father, in particular, takes on a new level of importance as the boy's awareness of the similarities between their genitals and urinary streams grows (Kleeman, 1966). Such awareness does not appear to be an isolated event. In their observations of children during the second year of life, Galenson and Roiphe (1974) were struck by the determination of toddlers to observe their parents' genitalia and elimination processes.

The recognition that his mother does not have a penis, whether through direct observation of her genitalia or that of a sibling or peer, facilitates the establishment of gender identity, assists the male toddler in the separation–individuation process, and produces castration anxiety. Castration anxiety is an observable aspect of life for young children which is best understood in the context of the toddler's limited cognitive ability and egocentricity. To the young boy, who has little capacity for rational thought, limited life experience and body awareness, the absence of a penis on someone as important to him as his mother or sister is bound to raise the possibility that the same thing could happen to this very special part of his own body.

In this developmental phase, as opposed to the next one, the father plays an important role in calming his son's castration fears.

> Optimally the father helps to minimize the boy's early castration anxiety and to stabilize core gender identity. He can reduce the influence of a mother's engulfing tendency as well as facilitate resolution of the rapprochement conflict, thereby rendering the castration threat implicit in these conflicts less noxious. As a male figure for identification, the father becomes still more important to the boy who is increasingly aware of being male and who looks for males with whom to identify; identifying with his father, it is easier for the boy to disidentify (Greenson, 1954) with his mother. Identification with the

father fosters a sense of masculinity and confidence in intact genitals and the boy's body image becomes more stable. (Tyson & Tyson, 1990, pp. 279–280)

Freud (1905) erroneously considered female sexual development to be the same as male development during the first 3 years of life. We now understand, by utilizing such concepts as core gender identity and the recognition of genital difference, that female sexuality has its own line of development which may be traced from birth onward. This new psychoanalytic theory of female sexuality, which was gradually evolving in the decades after Freud, may be explored in detail by the interested reader in the *Journal of the American Psychoanalytic Association, Supplement, Female Psychology*, which was published in 1976. Reference to articles from this supplement will be made throughout this volume.

As described by Roiphe and Galenson (1981), during the second year of life, girls, as well as boys, become aware of the anatomical differences between the sexes. Some of the girls in the study responded initially with what appeared to be sadness, anxiety, and withdrawal. Although speculative, since children in the second year of life do not have enough language development to communicate in detail what they are thinking, these findings are likely a reflection of the concreteness of the toddler's perceptions—a penis that can be seen and touched is preferable to a vagina which is less easily observed and defined. However, the girl's initial reaction to the absence of a penis must be placed in a broader developmental context in order to be fully understood, as was done by Tyson and Tyson (1990).

Observations of a little girl's reaction to the discovery of anatomical differences have often been interpreted as indicating a sense of castration or of penis envy (Mahler *et al.*, 1975; Roiphe & Galenson, 1981). Undoubtedly, these reactions occur, but we question whether they are the bedrock of normal female development, as Freud (1940) asserted. To understand the meaning of a girls' reaction, we must take account of her relationship to her parents, including the father's emotional (rather than sexual) availability as well as the mother's sense of her own femininity. When the mother–child relationship has been "good enough" and the mother is comfortable with her own femininity, the little girl may show surprise on discovering anatomical differences; she may even demonstrate a transitory fascination with or awe of the penis (Greenacre, 1953), be excited by and seek every opportunity to see a penis, and express wishes to have one. But at the same time she also has a sense of pride in being female. When father is libidinally available the fascination may lead to some early identification with him. Frequently penis fascination may be directed toward urinary functions, as when a little girl experiments with urinating standing up. This may express penis envy, or it may be an expression of envy of a boy's urinary prowess and a wish for similar bodily control. As Kestenberg (1976) noted, "the little girl 'wants a penis as a tool of control rather than an organ for pleasure' " (p. 223; see also Horney, 1924, pp. 260–261).

Cognitive Development

During the second and third year of life, cognitive development is transformed by the appearance of language. Essentially nonverbal at 1 year of age, by 3 years the young child has a vocabulary of several hundred words and the ability to communicate complex thoughts and feelings. Language not only transforms relationships but the intrapsychic world as well, for the child now has the ability to *symbolize*, to use words to represent inner and outer experience. Spitz's third psychic organizer, the "no," or negativism is the external indication of this profound intrapsychic transformation which so deeply characterizes human experience for the remainder of life.

According to Piaget, the toddler, at about 18 months, moves from the sensorimotor stage to that of concrete operations (ages 18 months to 12 years). Divided into two subphases, the preoperational period lasts from 18 months to 7 years. Language acquisition is a critical function during these years because it allows the toddler to substitute thoughts for actions. However, this newfound ability is limited by the toddler's lack of experience, egocentricity, and inability to abstract. Consequently, the toddler exaggerates his or her role in events, does not distinguish clearly between reality and fantasy, and cannot generalize.

Understanding the toddler's cognitive abilities and limitations is extremely important in the evaluation and treatment of children in this age group. Although most diagnostic efforts and therapeutic interventions center on the parents during the first 2 years of life, those children between 2 and 3 who have developed sufficient language ability may benefit from various forms of intervention directed primarily at them, including psychotherapy.

Evidence of Anality in Postanal Stages

The successful engagement of the major issues and conflicts of the anal stage of development has a profound effect upon personality development in the present and in the future. For instance,

> Disgust, orderliness, tidiness, dislike of dirty hands guard against the return of the repressed; punctuality, conscientiousness, and reliability appear as by

products of anal regularity; inclinations to save, to collect, give evidence of high anal evaluation displaced to other matters. In short, what takes place in this period is the far-reaching modification and transformation of the pregenital anal drive derivatives which—if kept within normal limits—supply the individual personality with a backbone of highly desirable, valuable qualities. (A. Freud, 1965, pp. 74–75)

Bathroom rituals and attitudes toward elimination obviously have their origins in the anal phase. So do the frequent references to anal activities and actions in conversations, jokes, and literature. Because of the pleasure associated with the anal area, anal activities are a normal part of sexual foreplay (as well as the primary focus in perversions). Attention to all of these areas by the psychotherapist will provide a pathway into the exploration of anal themes and conflicts.

CHAPTER 5

The Oedipal Phase (Ages 3–6)

INTRODUCTION

Freud based his theory of development during this phase on the myth of Oedipus. In Sophocles' tragedy, Oedipus unknowingly killed his father and married his mother. What we observe in young children between the ages of 3 and 6 is a persistent competition with the parent of the same sex for the attention and affection of the parent of the opposite sex (Freud, 1905). That is the essence of the Oedipal complex, nothing more, nothing less. However, that competition and desire must be understood from the vantage point of the physical and mental development of the 3-year-old, not the adult.

Children at this age are just beginning to think about the interactions between and among people, about relationships; particularly their own with the two most significant individuals in their lives, their mother and their father. This newfound capacity is the direct result of the attainment of object constancy (as discussed in Chapter Four), the ability to maintain mental representations of others in their absence. Because of it, the child can mentally engage his or her parents on a continuous basis, *fantasizing* about their interactions, manipulating the outcome in any way he or she chooses. This shift from dyadic (mother–child) to triadic (mother–father–child) fantasied and real relationships is evidence of a quantum leap forward in the child's ability to relate to others and the world; in other words, in object relationships (Loewald, 1985). The ability to engage the Oedipal complex rests squarely on these newly emergent ego functions which are the resultant of healthy preoedipal development.

In his attempt to describe the newly emerging vistas of the 3-year-old, Erikson (1963) described him or her as struggling with initiative versus guilt.

While autonomy concentrates on keeping potential rivals out, and therefore can lead to jealous rage most often directed against encroachments by younger siblings, initiative brings with it anticipatory rivalry with those who have been there first and may, therefore, occupy with their superior equipment the field toward which one's initiative is directed. Infantile jealousy and rivalry, those often embittered and yet essentially futile attempts at demarcating a sphere of unquestioned privilege now come to a climax in a final contest for a favored position with the mother; the usual failure leads to resignation, guilt and anxiety. The child indulges in fantasies of being a giant and a tiger, but in his dreams he runs in terror for dear life. (pp. 255–256)

Some of the child's fantasies and preoccupations are sexual, but again, not in the adult sense. In order to understand the nature of sexuality in the Oedipal-aged child, let us first briefly review the developmental line of sexual identity formation during the first 3 years of life and then explore the concept of infantile sexuality.

As discussed in Chapters Three and Four, during the first 18 months of life children develop *core gender identity.* Then, during the second and third year of life, they learn that there are two different kinds of genitalia and that they, as a male or female, possess one of the two. Thus, the child enters the Oedipal phase with a strong but concrete and rudimentary awareness of sexual difference.

INFANTILE SEXUALITY

The Case of "Little Hans"

Infantile sexuality refers to the nature of sexual thought and action in childhood *as experienced and understood by the child.* Some adults, unfamiliar with the essence of development of cognitive and emotional processes in early childhood, assume incorrectly that the child has the same physical and emotional sexual experiences as they do. In order to understand the similarities and differences between infantile and adult sexuality, let us examine Freud's case of "Little Hans," more formally called "The Analysis of a Phobia in a Five-Year-Old Boy" (1909). Freud became acquainted with Hans when his father, a student of Freud's, sought help for his son's fear of horses, a phobia which was quite restricting in the Vienna of 1909. As Hans's father brought material from the boy to "the Professor," Freud would make suggestions which the father then carried out. In his case report, Freud gave many vivid illustrations of the nature of the infantile sexual mind, examples which have been confirmed innumerable times by parents and other observers of children in the last 80 years. Although the case material is about a boy, the same kind of sexual curiosity, actions, and interactions with parents is observed in girls.

Curiosity about the Nature of the Genitals. Not quite 3 years old, Hans was "showing a quite peculiarly lively interest in that portion of his body which he used to describe as his 'widdler' " (Freud, 1909, p. 7).

Hans was becoming preoccupied with the highly pleasurable sensations which he could produce in his penis and nowhere else in his body. His interest in his penis caused him to become intensely curious about the presence or absence of widdlers in the world around him.

HANS: "Mummy, have you got a widdler too?"

MOTHER: "Of course. Why?"

HANS: "I was only just thinking." (p. 7)

At the same age, Hans saw a cow being milked. "Oh look!" he said, "there's milk coming out of its widdler!" Several months later he saw some water being let out of an engine. "Oh, look," he said, "the engine's widdling. Where's it got its widdler?" After a while he added reflectively "a dog and a horse have widdlers, a table and a chair haven't" (p. 9).

Freud did not have the benefit of Piaget's theory of cognitive development, as we do, to help him understand the nature of the young child's mind. But he clearly demonstrated Hans's concrete attempts to grapple with the animate versus the inanimate and more specifically to understand which animals, human and otherwise, had penises or body parts which resembled them. Hans's thinking, certainly confused and humorous from an adult standpoint, is quite normal and phase-appropriate for a 3-year-old.

The Inseparable Connection between the Thirst for Knowledge and Sexual Curiosity about the Parents. As Hans moved through the Oedipal years his sexual curiosity focused more and more on those individuals who were closest to him, his parents. Hans first struggled to discover what his parents' genitals were like and then began, in action and thought, to attempt to engage his mother in sexual play with him.

HANS: "Daddy, have you got a widdler too?"

FATHER: "Yes, of course."

HANS: "But I've never seen it when you were undressing." (Freud, 1909, p. 9)

Hans was still puzzled by his mother's genitals and continued to watch her like a hawk. One night while she was undressing for bed they had the following interchange.

MOTHER: "What are you staring like that for?"

HANS: "I was only looking to see if you've got a widdler too."

MOTHER: "Of course, don't you know that?"

HANS: "No, I thought you were so big you'd have a widdler like a horse."
(pp. 9–10)

In his expectation of bigness, Hans displays another aspect of infantile sexuality, a preoccupation with size. The Oedipal-aged child is beginning to recognize the disadvantage of being small in a world controlled by large adults and to focus on the idea, which some men and women never abandon, that when it comes to penises size, and not function, is all important.

Infantile Masturbation. When Hans was 3½ years old Freud noted, "Meanwhile his interest in his widdler was by no means a purely theoretical one; as might be expected, it also impelled him to touch his member" (Freud, 1909, p. 7). Children learn of the unique pleasures which are produced by stimulating their genitals from infancy onward, from their own manipulation and as a result of being diapered and bathed by others.

By the time Hans was 4 years old and an old hand at self-stimulation he actively turned to the seduction of his mother.

"This morning Hans was given his usual daily bath by his mother and afterwards dried and powdered. As she was powdering around his penis and taking care not to touch it, Hans said: 'Why don't you put your finger there?'"

MOTHER: "Because that'd be piggish."

HANS: "What's that? Piggish? Why?"

MOTHER: "Because it's not proper."

HANS: (*laughing*) "But it's great fun." (p. 19)

As those of us who treat young children know, the physical act of masturbation, in children (as in adults) is accompanied by elaborate fantasies. Hans was no exception.

Hans came to his father early one morning because he was frightened. When asked what was wrong, he said: "I put my finger to my widdler just a very little. I saw Mummy quite naked in her chemise, and she let me see her widdler. I showed Grete (a girlfriend), my Grete, what Mummy was doing and showed her my widdler. Then I took my hand away from my widdler quick." When the father asked about the mother's chemise, Hans said: "She was in her chemise, but the chemise was so short that I saw her widdler." (p. 32) The fantasy occurred soon after Hans was told women did not have widdlers. He obviously had not accepted the fact. Grete was involved because he wished to show her his penis. If mother showed her widdler, it would be all right for him to show his. Children of this age do masturbate to orgasm, in the sense of a rhythmic pulsation of the genitals with intense feeling, but without the release of semen in the boy, obviously.

Knowledge of these developmental processes can be extremely helpful to the clinician in attempting to determine if a young child has been sexually abused or not. Oedipal-aged children do fantasize about sexual involvement with adults. However, as with Little Hans, these fantasies are limited by the child's physical and intellectual immaturity. When the child talks about activities which can only occur in the sexually mature body, the diagnostician can strongly suspect that sexual abuse has occurred. Examples would be descriptions of oral, vaginal, or anal penetration by the penis and ejaculation of semen because penetration and ejaculation are totally foreign concepts to the young child.

Many sexually abused children will spontaneously talk about or play out the abuse. Others can be encouraged to talk about it by trained members of sexual abuse teams. Whenever possible, suspected abuse should be confirmed by physical examination.

OEDIPAL DEVELOPMENT IN THE BOY

Although the nature of infantile sexuality is essentially the same in boys and in girls, there are major differences between the sexes which must be considered separately. Many of Freud's ideas on male development have been confirmed and elaborated. However, his theory of female sexuality has been largely discarded and replaced because it was an erroneous extrapolation of the male model which described femininity in negative terms.

During infancy the preoedipal mother is at the center of the boy's world as she provides for his physical needs, enhances his psychological individuation, and teaches him about the world. Building upon his dawning understanding of sexual difference and curiosity about male–female relationships our budding Oedipus gradually becomes interested in his mother as a sexual being and begins to include her in his own infantile sexual world. His ingrained sense of maleness (Edgcumbe & Burgner, 1975) and his growing awareness that his father has a relationship with his mother which is very different from his own (for example, they sleep together while he sleeps alone) gradually draws him into competition with his father for his mother's attention and affections. These hostile, competitive feelings begin to produce internal conflict because they intrude upon the deep feelings of love for father which preceded them.

The father's ongoing presence (Tyson, 1982) and reaction to his son's hostility is critically important in determining the course of the boy's development. If he is tolerant and accepting without being either seductive or punitive, the father will provide an atmosphere in which his son can struggle with his conflicting thoughts and feelings utilizing the limited, but sufficient, psychological resources available to him. And struggle he does, particularly with his fantasies. The boy's wishes to displace and attack, even to kill his father, are frightening as well as gratifying. His progenitor is much bigger and more powerful than he and on numerous occasions has used his power to restrict or punish. Thus, every wish to attack the father becomes increasingly associated with fear and an expectation of retaliation. The child's limited ability to sharply distinguish fantasy from reality makes his hostile wishes and fear of retaliation all the more threatening. For these reasons, it is most important—in regard to both boys and girls—that Oedipal bravado and competitiveness, particularly with the parent of the same sex, not be punished. Broad limits on behavior obviously need to be set, but the time-limited, phase-specific Oedipal challenge, so essential to normal developmental progression, should be understood and accepted. Indeed, the healthy parent, sure of his or her own sexuality, will find the pseudochallenge and the wish to be emulated and displaced, highly enjoyable.

As his investment in his penis becomes more focused and valued, and through masturbation closely tied to his fantasies about love for his mother and competition with his father, the boy begins to experience castration anxiety; essentially the fear that his father's retaliation will take away his maleness. In the concrete mind of the child this danger is not symbolic but real, heightened by the erroneous but understandable belief that females had penises and somehow lost them. This idea is not the fanciful production of the adult mind; rather it is repeatedly thrust upon us by both boys and girls in this age group. For example, I was recently told the following anecdote by the mother of a 3-year-old boy who had just begun to attend a nursery school which had one bathroom with several toilets that were used by both sexes. When asked why he was touching his penis so frequently, the boy replied that he was checking to see if it was still there. He had noticed at school that the girls had lost their penises and he did not want to lose his. Realistically absurd, this idea is perfectly logical to the concrete, egocentric mind of the 3-year-old.

However, because of their innate curiosity and depth of attachment to their mothers, boys also admire the female body. They are deeply curious about the female genitals and envious of the women's breasts and ability to have babies (Ross, 1975). When these thoughts are put into words, as they sometimes are early in the Oedipal phase, they threaten parental comfort about their son's masculinity and may result in a refer-ral. As always, a thorough diagnostic assessment should be done, but the clinician should be aware of the developmental appropriateness of such wishes at about age 3. In most boys these wishes are quickly repressed and rarely verbalized again.

Masturbation is a normal, necessary Oedipal experience which inten-sifies fantasy production by adding the component of intense genital pleasure, and later assists in the "resolution" of the Oedipal complex by heightening castration anxiety. The typical masturbatory fantasy at this age has not changed since the days of Little Hans; it involves sexual play with mother but not penetration or ejaculation. These components of male sexuality do not become apparent until adolescence, stimulated by the biological events surrounding puberty.

The Oedipal complex is gradually "resolved" (Freud, 1924) as the fear of castration becomes stronger than the sexual wishes for the mother. This process is aided by the boy's gradual recognition of his relative weakness and impotence in a world controlled by adults and by his growing desire to be like his father and other men and boys. In the end, aided by the internalization of the superego (a subject we will consider in Chapter Six), he decides on the following, wise course of action: "If you can't beat 'em, join 'em." With this goal in mind, he turns his attention away from his intense fantasy world and his penis, away from his mother and girls, whom he loudly devalues, and enters latency; there to learn what his father, friends, and culture consider to be masculine.

OEDIPAL DEVELOPMENT IN THE GIRL

As previously described, during the first 18 months of life every girl develops a core gender identity, a basic sense of femaleness on which her future sexual development rests. This idea, a cornerstone concept in the new theory of female sexuality, is very different from Freud's idea that girls and boys had the same, essentially male, orientation prior to the Oedipus phase. He postulated that all children conceptualized the penis as their genitalia, consequently, girls were placed in the painful, inferior position of determining what had happened to them, what had produced their castrated state?

In their studies of sexual development in the second and third years of life, Galenson and Roiphe (1976) noticed that many of the girls they studied did experience a temporary affective change in the form of sad-ness or withdrawal following the discovery of the penis.

Comparisons between the penis and the vagina confront the preoedipal girl with a very difficult task, considering her limited cognitive abilities; because her own genital organ is not as easily seen or conceptualized as the penis and testicles. "Something" versus "nothing" is the initial mental concern of the 2-year-old as she struggles to understand the nature of her genitalia. Gradually, this simplistic idea is replaced by an awareness that her genital organ is complex, partly internal and the source of powerful pleasurable sensations (Kestenberg, 1968). Another reason for the girl's focus on the entire genital area—labia, clitoris, and vagina—rather than the clitoris *per se* is the nature of genital sensation which is thought to be more diffuse; experienced as emanating from the entire genital area as opposed to being focused in the head of the penis, as it is in the boy. This idea that the girl experiences her genitals as diffuse, complex, and partly internal is much more meaningful than Freud's belief that she has little awareness of her sexual organs prior to adolescence. Indeed, it has been suggested that the confrontation of this difficult conceptual task so early in life may be an explanation for the emergence of feminine intuition, sensitivity, and awareness. By contrast, boys are not nearly as intellectually or emotionally stimulated by the relatively simple task of looking between their legs to see what is there.

There is one additional, very painful, step which the girl must take in order to enter the Oedipal phase. Unlike the boy, she must partially abandon her deep attachment to the mother and transfer her sexually determined interest and affection to the father. Once this is accomplished, the girl's Oedipal development proceeds on a course similar to the boy's. She becomes increasingly interested in her father's body and desires to possess and explore it for her own sexual purposes. She recognizes that her mother occupies a unique place of physical and psychological closeness to her father and tries to displace her. The desire to displace the mother conflicts painfully with the deep, abiding love for her which has been present since infancy.

Eventually, the girl resolves the Oedipal complex in the same manner as the boy. Because of her love for her mother and the fear of retaliation by the bigger, powerful parent, she gradually mutes her sexual desires and fantasies and, through identification with her mother and other important females in her life, plunges into the latency-age task of expanding her understanding of what it means to be female.

THE NEGATIVE OEDIPAL COMPLEX

Because the child has loving feelings toward both parents, he or she also experiences a negative (or reverse of the more prominent, positive)

Oedipal complex. In this constellation of fantasies and actions, the child competes with the parent of the opposite sex for the affections and attention of the parent of the same sex. This is not surprising in view of the depth of attachment which children experience toward both parents in early childhood. The negative Oedipal complex is a constant theme in the child's emotional life, helping him or her maintain a loving relationship with the parent of the same sex in the face of ongoing challenge and competitiveness. It also functions as a template for the psychological expression and containment of homosexual feelings.

TYPICAL OEDIPAL PHENOMENA— THEIR MEANING AND SUGGESTED ADULT RESPONSE

Fears, Phobias, and Nightmares—the Infantile Neurosis

The child at age 3 or 4 begins to have fears, phobias, and nightmares. Suddenly he or she is afraid of the dark, afraid to go upstairs alone. The shadow at the window becomes a ghost trying to get in; the open closet door an invitation to the monster who lurks there to explode into the bedroom and devour his young victim. Sleep, no longer peaceful, is frequently interrupted by nightmares, typically of someone with evil intent speeding toward the helpless child who suddenly cannot move to escape.

These are normal phenomena at this stage of development, and are indications that the child is actively engaged in the Oedipal conflict and resorting to symptom formation to manage the too powerful sexual and aggressive thoughts and feelings which flood his or her mind. The ability to form these neurotic symptoms, which indicates a major advance in ego development, particularly in the use of the defense mechanisms of repression, projection, and displacement, is called the *infantile neurosis* (Freud, 1918). The phobic symptoms of the Oedipal phase have the same construction as phobic neuroses which occur in later life; but unlike their adult counterparts, the infantile versions are signs of developmental progression, heralding the engagement of the Oedipal complex and the emergence, for the first time in childhood, of the ability to use sophisticated defense mechanisms to control internal conflict.

The Oedipal phase is the only time in life when persistent fears, phobias, and nightmares are considered to be normal. Their presence in other stages of development, such as late latency or adolescence, is an indication of pathology, calling for diagnostic intervention. This is a good example of the principle stated in Chapter One, that what is normal at one phase of development may be abnormal at another. When neurotic symptomatology does occur later in childhood or adulthood, the clinician should consider that all neuroses stem from unresolved Oedipal conflict. A careful developmental history will facilitate an understanding of the internal and environmental factors which precipitated the formation of the neuroses and an awareness of the nature of Oedipal thought and feeling will assist in deciphering the presentation of the internal conflicts behind the neurotic symptoms in the therapeutic setting.

Knowledge of these developmental principles will also help the clinician understand the Oedipal child diagnostically and therapeutically, and advise parents and other adults about how to interact with children in this age group. Parents should not attempt to talk the child out of his or her fears or give credence to the idea that the ghosts, goblins, or monsters are real but controllable. Rather they should reassure the child that they will be available as a continual source of comfort and security. As the child moves into latency, the symptoms of the infantile neurosis diminish on their own, their disappearance indicating the "resolution" of the Oedipal complex and the internalization of the superego.

Size Comparisons

Oedipal-aged children are preoccupied with size comparisons. They are just becoming aware of the power connected with being big, something they lack in themselves and envy in their parents. Children of this age will typically stand next to an adult and compare heights or place their hand next to a grown-up's and measure the difference. Frequently, they will comment, painfully or angrily, with remarks such as "Why are you so big?" or "When I grow up you're going to be small." Sometimes the anger engendered by such comparisons will be translated into physical attacks, occasionally thinly disguised as accidental or playful, aimed at the genitals of the parent of the same sex. Parents should neither belittle nor encourage the size comparisons because they are serious business to the child, the source of considerable pain and anger. With an understanding of what is occurring, the parent can sensitively accept the child's recriminations and anticipate the physical attacks which may follow.

The Misinterpretation of Adult Interventions

Because Oedipal-aged children are so preoccupied with hostile impulses toward adults and the expectation of retaliation, they *mis-*

interpret the intention of many adult actions toward them, interpreting them as punitive or seductive. Examples are medical and surgical procedures and the use of enemas and suppositories. Because of this, *elective* medical and surgical procedures should be avoided at this phase of development. Regardless of how sensitive the adults performing the intervention may be, the child will distort their intent and see their actions as an attack, a retaliation for the child's fantasized preoccupation with the wish to be grown up and displace adults from positions of power and control. These feelings are heightened if the genital area is involved. Even when the genital area is not involved, the child will express concerns about the genitals; for example, the refusal of children in this age group to remove their underwear prior to a tonsillectomy. Enemas and suppositories are also invasive procedures which produce highly stimulating sensations as well as painful ones. Rarely needed from a medical standpoint, their use, particularly by parents, is interpreted by the child as an act of vengeance or seduction. For these same reasons physicians who are parents should not consistently examine or treat their children. The roles of parent and physician are best managed by the child when performed in a consistent, caring manner by different adults.

Masturbation

As previously described, masturbation is a normal phenomenon during the Oedipal phase and an integral part of the developmental process. Freud's (1923) discovery of infantile masturbation was greeted by shock, disbelief, and dismay. The clinician will find similar reactions in some parents in the present and should be prepared to deal with them empathetically. They are often based on unresolved conflicts about sexuality which are stimulated by the openness and intensity of the child's sexual behavior, which must be denied or diminished. Even at this age most masturbation is done in private but occasionally it will take place in public, or in the parents' presence, for the specific purpose of involving them à la Little Hans. As with most aspects of normal sexual behavior, parents should neither encourage nor criticize masturbatory activity. On those occasions when it occurs in inappropriate settings the child should be gently asked to stop, and informed that such activities are usually performed in the privacy of one's room. Compulsive masturbation at this age is usually a sign that the child has been overstimulated sexually, and is unable to manage sexual preoccupations primarily through thoughts, feelings, and fantasies.

Sexual Curiosity

Oedipal-aged children are intensely curious about sexuality in themselves and others. Consequently, questions about sex abound as do attempts to initiate physical contact with the parents.

Sexual questions should be answered honestly and straightforwardly in language which the child can understand, the response limited to the question being asked and not expanded into a lecture. For example, Question: "Daddy, where do babies come from?" Answer: "From inside of the mommy." If the child is satisfied, the question may stop at this point; if not others will follow, building on the previous one. Question: "How do they get out?" Answer: "There's a special opening between the mother's legs." Satisfied response: "Oh."

Volunteering more than the child asks or using the adult body to educate by demonstrating body parts or functions may flood the child with more information or feeling than he or she can comfortably integrate because of limited cognitive capacities and ability to contain powerful feelings.

It is most important for adults to understand that the Oedipal-aged child has neither the body nor the mind to understand adult sexuality in a factual, experiential, or emotional sense. Oedipal "resolution" is based, in part, on the comfortable management of powerful sexual feelings, some factual information, and numerous misconceptions. In other words, adults facilitate the developmental process best by not imposing their own bodies or mental set upon the child. The ability to understand adult sexuality develops later, increasing in latency and taking a quantum leap forward in adolescence because of the attainment of a sexually mature body and the development of the capacity for abstract thinking. For these reasons, there is a definite need for formal sex education in the schools beginning in the late elementary grades and extending into junior and senior high school. Children in these age groups should be provided information which resonates with their level of physical, cognitive, and social maturity. For instance, in the late elementary grades, the focus would be on the physical and psychological changes surrounding puberty. In junior high school, the emphasis would shift to dating, sexual relationships, contraception, sexually transmitted diseases, and moral attitudes. In senior high school (and in college) courses on marriage, parenthood, and normal and pathological child and adult development would complete the preparation for adult life. Formal sexual education in the schools should be supplemented throughout by parental readiness to guide the child/adolescent toward a comfortable, responsible attitude about normal adolescent and young adult sexual activity.

Attempts to gain sexual information and experience through actions are nearly constant on the child's part. Displaying their genitals, parading around the house nude, climbing into the parents' bed, observing the adults closely in the acts of dressing or showering, initiating frequent bodily contact, particularly in the genital area, are some of the ways Oedipal-aged children involve their parents in their sexual fantasies and preoccupations. When parents allow these interactions to occur *on a regular basis*, they stimulate sexual thoughts and feelings which the child cannot understand, integrate, or master. Frequently, such overstimulation leads to symptom formation.

The practicing child therapist is repeatedly presented with examples of unwitting or unconscious overstimulation on the part of parents. A young father, who was in therapy for unrelated matters, described his great pleasure and pride in taking showers with his 3-year-old daughter. He loved the physical closeness which existed between them and wanted his daughter to grow up without a sense of shame about the human body. This attitude continued until the day when she, just 3½ years old and crotch high to him, grabbed his penis. "Daddy," she said, clutching his penis with glee, "this is *so big!*" That was the last shower they took together.

A second, more pathologic example came to light in the treatment of an 8-year-old girl who had severe nightmares and phobias. A detailed history revealed that she had frequently observed her parents having intercourse by coming into their bedroom at night and standing at the foot of their bed. After I explained to the parents about the relationship between sexual overstimulation and phobias and nightmares, they agreed to put a lock on the bedroom door. As a result of this intervention and the psychotherapeutic work with the child, the nightmares gradually diminished until they suddenly reappeared, following a period of several weeks in which the parents "forgot" to lock the bedroom door. The same family sent me a postcard from a European trip they took with my patient and her siblings. The postcard pictured the famous redlight district of Amsterdam and contained the notation, "the girls really enjoyed seeing this."

THE PLIGHT OF THE SINGLE PARENT

Separation and divorce complicate the developmental process for the Oedipal-aged child who functions best when he or she has two parents who love each other, set appropriate limits, and understand what the child is experiencing. However, children raised in single-parent situations can successfully progress through the Oedipal phase with some parental help and understanding. Single parents should facilitate the child's access to one another on a regular basis and refrain from criticism of the absent parent. They should not use the child as a source of solace and comfort for their own loss by taking the child into bed or elevating him or her to the role of pseudo-spouse. Modesty should continue to be maintained and limits set. Finally, the child should not be exposed to parental involvement in causal dating or sexual situations. Potential stepparents should be introduced gradually, never as a replacement for the biological parent, when the relationship is likely to be significant and lasting.

If the parent of the same sex as the child is not involved and there is no acceptable replacement, the child will use whoever is available in the environment, be it a neighbor, teacher, parent of a friend, or relative, as an object for identification and competition. Whenever appropriate, these relationships should be facilitated by the parent of the opposite sex. In addition, the child will resort to fantasy and imagination to create an Oedipal competitor. Obviously, this is a difficult situation for the child and is not conducive to an easy resolution of Oedipal issues.

THE TRANSITION TO LATENCY

Because of the absence of an organized superego, the Oedipal child is free to entertain sexual and aggressive fantasies without fear of internal incrimination. However, as these thoughts and feelings become increasingly focused on the parents and are rejected or greeted with disdain or punishment, they begin to be questioned. Gradually, the child begins to mute his or her Oedipal strivings and to adhere to parental expectations because of "the triple threat of bodily harm, narcissistic injury, and loss of love . . . increasingly the child becomes aware that the parents not only enforce behavioral standards but themselves live by a set of moral and ethical codes." As these codes are idealized, he or she constructs an "internal morality in identification with the rather concretely idealized parental moral standards" (Tyson & Tyson, 1990, pp. 217–218). The gradual strengthening of this inner voice pushes the child away from the preoccupation with incestuous wishes and toward their repression and disavowal, thus beginning the process of Oedipal resolution and the internalization of the superego as a consistent presence, a powerful inner voice which dramatically changes the nature of thought, feeling, and action in the next phase of development—latency.

CHAPTER 6

Latency (Ages 6–11)

When I think of elementary school children, I see them rushing and tumbling at recess, balancing on railings, climbing, sliding, swinging with zest, chanting their rhymes, sucking lollipops, comic books in their hands, tearing around chasing one another. I hear the sound of roller skates on the pavements, hopscotch chalked on the sidewalks, the girls skipping ropes to chants. (Elizabeth Bremner Kaplan, 1965, p. 220)

INTRODUCTION

The latency phase of development encompasses the years 6 to 11, "latent" in the sense that this is an interval of relative calm between the intense psychological turmoil of the Oedipal phase and the profound biopsychological upheaval of adolescence. *Relative* is the key word since although the comparisons between the external appearance of growth and development during latency and the Oedipal phase and adolescence are accurate, major developmental advances occur during these years. Freud (1905) introduced the term, relating the beginning of latency to a psychological event, the resolution of the Oedipal complex, and its end to a maturational one, the occurrence of puberty.

Normal latency begins as the Oedipal child, increasingly aware that he or she cannot win the dangerous conflict, gradually replaces the desire to challenge the parent of the same sex with the wish to be like him or her. The transition is facilitated by the formation of a new psychic structure—the superego. Built upon the introjected authority of the parents, this constantly vigilant monitor guards against the conscious consideration and enjoyment of unbridled sexual and aggressive wishes and fantasies. Using other terminology, the reality principle and secondary process thinking gradually gain ascendancy over the pleasure principle and primary process thinking (Freud, 1924b). As the ego and superego gradually gain control over the drives, dramatic changes take place in action and thought.

DIVISIONS OF LATENCY

Bornstein (1951) divided latency into two phases, early (5½ to 8) and late (8 to 10/11). Early latency is a time of transition. As the child represses the Oedipal complex, adjusts to the restrictions of the superego, and moves out of the nuclear family into the community, he or she is often tense, anxious, and ambivalent, given to frequent mood swings and regressive behavior.

By contrast, late latency is in the normal child a time of smooth growth and development. A brief moment of tranquillity referred to as the golden age of childhood, it is characterized by comfortable relationships with peers and adults and an intense interest in exploring the world and learning new skills.

Shapiro and Perry (1976) suggested that at age 7, plus or minus 1, there is a convergence of maturational factors, particularly in the central nervous system, which partially accounts for the significant cognitive and behavioral changes which are observed at midlatency. They include the emergence of concrete operations (Piaget) and secondary process thinking, increased control of impulses, and the comfortable repression of the active fantasy life of the Oedipal stage.

THE DEVELOPMENTAL TASKS OF LATENCY

Like all other developmental phases, latency is characterized by the presence of several issues, unique to these years, which must be engaged and mastered if normal developmental progression is to occur. They are the consolidation of the superego; the elaboration of masculine or feminine identifications, thus continuing and expanding the developmental line of sexual identity; the formation of significant peer relationships; and the acquisition of new mental and physical skills and interests.

Superego Formation

In 1914, Sigmund Freud first introduced the idea of an agency of the mind, which watches over the ego and compares it to an ideal standard. The main impetus to the formation of this judgmental aspect of the personality is parental criticism, expanded as the child grows by education, training, and cultural standards. Elaborating on these ideas in 1921, Freud spoke of the feelings of triumph and pleasure which are experienced when thought and action coincide with the expectations of the conscience.

In *The Ego and the Id*, Freud (1923) presented the structure theory (id, ego, and superego) and related the formation of the superego to the resolution of the Oedipal complex and the beginning of latency; postulating the need for a psychic agency which would ensure that unbridled sexual and aggressive fantasies could no longer be consciously entertained without experiencing the painful affect of guilt. The formation of the superego acts as a positive stimulant to further development by freeing the child of Oedipal preoccupations and becoming the vehicle for the internalization of morality.

Although the superego becomes organized in latency, the process of formation may be traced through the preoedipal and Oedipal years, particularly in relationship to parental limit-setting activities which the child internalizes; for instance, the toddler actively integrating the parental "No" (Spitz) and using it to judge his or her own and others' actions.

In early latency, the superego is experienced as a foreign body. Primitive and demanding, it is unreliable and accounts in part for the frequent moodiness and regression observed during these years. By late latency, it becomes more integrated and moderate, providing some of the basis for the calm rationality and self-confidence which characterize the years between 8 and 11.

Once the superego is in place, it becomes the major source of self-esteem, replacing the parents. These "loving and beloved" aspects of the superego are just as important to healthy development as the control of thought and action (Schafer, 1960). The major mechanics involved in superego formation are introjection and identification (Sandler, 1960). Through introjection—the introject has the capacity to substitute in whole or in part for the real object as a source of narcissistic identification—the relationship to the real objects, the parents, is maintained and perpetuated; but their function as prohibitor, judge, and source of self-esteem is diminished. Through identification the self is modified so that it corresponds to a greater or lesser degree with the object (the parents) as perceived by the ego.

The internalization of the superego and the repression of Oedipal strivings and competitiveness have a powerful effect on the latency-aged child's relationship with the parents. No longer consciously preoccupied with stimulating and disturbing fantasies, he or she can manage a calmer, more modulated relationship which is based on mutual interests and realistic consideration. Competitiveness is replaced by identification and admiration, time is spent together enjoyably, and a sense of calm, "mature" mutuality prevails. Latency is the golden age of childhood for the parents as well as for the child.

THE EMERGENCE OF THE CAPACITY FOR FRIENDSHIP

The representation of Oedipal strivings, the growth of the ego, particularly the capacity to control impulses and delay gratification, and the movement out of the home into the broader community are all necessary prerequisites for the emergence of the capacity to form friendships.

Definition. For Freud (1921) friendship was a form of love stemming from the same source as sexual love.

> We do not separate from this—what in any case has its share in the name "love"—on the one hand, self love, and on the other, love of parents and children, friendship and love for humanity in general, and also devotion to concrete objects and to abstract ideas. (p. 90)

In the relationship between the sexes impulses "force their way toward sexual union, but in other circumstances *they are diverted from this aim and are prevented from reaching it*" (italics added, pp. 90–91). So an important distinction between love and friendship is the aim-inhibited expression of the impulses in friendships. But human beings are aggressive as well as loving.

> As a result, their neighbor is for them not only a potential helper or sexual object, but also someone who tempts them to satisfy their aggressiveness on him, to exploit his capacity for work without compensation, to use him sexually without his consent, to seize his possessions, to humiliate him, to cause him pain, to torture and to kill him. (Freud, 1930, p. 111)

Based on these and other considerations, Nemiroff and I (1985) formulated the following definition of friendship: "friendship is an extrafamilial object relationship based on mutuality, equality and freedom of choice, in which the expression of sexual and aggressive impulses is predominantly aim inhibited" (p. 75).

By limiting friendships to extrafamilial settings, this definition rules out many important relationships in which friendly feelings occur, such as those between parents and children, lovers, and siblings; because the essential nature of these interactions is either the direct expression of sexual impulses (lovers) or the absence of choice (parents, children, and siblings).

The Precursors of Friendship

Rangell (1963) suggested that friendly feelings have their roots in the gratifying relationship between infant and mother. Then, during the preoedipal and Oedipal years, friendly feelings begin to be focused on individuals outside of the nuclear family, but these relationships are "transient, mostly nonspecific, internally directed, and self oriented, of use primarily for the consolidation of *inner* psychic development" (p. 116).

However, with the resolution of the Oedipal complex "love, which has now reached an intense developmental peak, can be diluted and mitigated, objects (again) displaced, and aims inhibited and less than directly sought" (Rangell, 1963, p. 17). Because of these events, the formation of the superego, the increased capacity for sublimation, and the movement out of the home into the community and the school, all of the prerequisites for the formation of true friendships are in place by early latency. Because these new relationships are such an integral part of latency experience, they significantly affect the progression along a number of developmental lines, particularly the elaboration of sexual identity and play.

Elaboration of Sexual Identity and Peer Relationships

Tracing the developmental line of sexual identity through the first three developmental phases, we noted the establishment of core gender identity (oral), followed by the recognition of genital difference between the sexes (anal), which set the stage for the preoccupation with the role of sexuality in relationships during the Oedipal stage. Now, during latency, masculinity and femininity are considered within the environment outside of the home, adding a subjective cultural dimension.

Because of the need to maintain the repression and avoidance of Oedipal interests which are now prohibited by the superego, the latency focus is on same sex preoccupations and the active avoidance of the opposite sex. Boys play with boys and hate girls and vice versa. In the rush to be more masculine or feminine, nearly every activity is assigned to one sex or the other. This subjective determination is influenced primarily by family values and peers. For example, in a family in which father, grandfather, and uncles play classical guitar, a latency-aged boy's interest in the guitar may be very "masculine"; in another, nonmusical family, such an interest might be considered "feminine."

This arbitrary division into masculine or feminine is very strong in the peer group where there is constant vigilance against the demonstration of interest in the opposite sex and the desire to participate in activities and games which have been assigned to the "despised" opposition. Broader cultural attitudes toward masculinity or femininity are added through interest in and identification with figures from sports, literature, and the popular media. This normal, phase-limited need to exaggerate the differences between the sexes begins to disappear during preadolescence and is gone forever during adolescence, replaced by the biologically driven need for heterosexual interaction.

Despite the strong effort to avoid heterosexual interests and actions, masturbation is an integral part of the life of most latency-aged children (Clower, 1976). Consisting of the direct or indirect stimulation of the genitals, sometimes to climax, it occurs less frequently than during the Oedipal phase and adolescence and is sometimes devoid of conscious fantasy. Children in this age group are particularly secretive about their masturbation and are very reluctant to discuss it, even with a trusted therapist.

Peer relationships play a critical role during latency not only in the elaboration of sexual identity but also in the gradual movement out of the nuclear family into the community and in the alteration of psychic structure and drive discharge. The attitudes and standards of peers and significant adults, such as teachers, add a vital balancing component to the superego while at the same time providing a nonincestuous framework for the discharge of sexual and aggressive impulses through discussion and group activities.

An understanding of the nature of peer relationships during latency has great clinical relevance, particularly diagnostically. The latency peer group acts as a cruel but accurate triage unit, accepting those children who manifest the ability to psychologically separate from parents and engage the developmental tasks of latency, and rejecting those who are regressed and immature. Consequently, acceptance by the same sex peer group is one of the best gauges of psychological health during latency, and rejection is a frequent indication of pathology and a very common presenting symptom.

Understanding the tendency to avoid the opposite sex and naturally segregate into same sex groups is also very important for educators, parents, and professionals as evidenced by the following example from my experience as a school consultant.

Late one afternoon, I received a frantic call for "help" from an elementary school principal. She had just tried, unsuccessfully, to contain a shouting match between a third grade teacher and the parents of one of her students who were arguing over the discipline imposed on Johnny. What should she do now? It appeared that the teacher had asked her class to line up by twos to go to the auditorium for assembly. The students quickly scrambled to find their friends and sorted themselves into same-sex pairs—except for two, Johnny and a girl! Johnny refused to stand next to his assigned partner, let alone hold her hand, as instructed by the teacher. After several refusals to comply with her orders, the teacher called Johnny a disobedient little boy and sent him to the principal's office. Later she sent a note to Johnny's home describing the incident and her reaction to it. In the meeting among the principal, teacher, and parents which was requested by the parents, the unsuccessful discussion about teacher insensitivity versus the need for discipline ended in a shouting match. If the teacher had understood developmental theory she would have allowed Johnny to straggle along, alone, at the end of the line and avoided the entire incident. Educational and parental practices and therapeutic technique work when they incorporate expressions of the normal developmental process, rather than oppose them.

ADJUSTMENT TO SCHOOL AND FORMAL LEARNING

Just as acceptance by the latency-aged peer group is a good indicator of normal developmental progression, so is successful adjustment to the elementary school setting. The school's role as assessor of early development is one of its most important functions since it is the first social agency outside of the nuclear family which intensively and realistically evaluates the child. Protected within the cocoon of the nuclear family from the intense scrutiny of society for the first 5 or 6 years of life, the school-aged child must now demonstrate the ability to function independently within a complex, goal-oriented setting.

The transition from home to school may seem simple since most children accomplish it without great difficulty, but successful adjustment indicates that development is progressing normally along multiple developmental lines. The child who adjusts to kindergarten or first grade must be able to control his or her body, which includes bowel and bladder control and the ability to sit still; demonstrate the cognitive maturity for readiness activities, the forerunners of reading and writing; separate from parents and be able to relate to strange adults, sharing their interest and affection with others; relate to peers and accept the rough-and-tumble interactions within the peer group; and accomplish all this with a considerable degree of impulse control and a minimum degree of regression.

As the elementary school years progress and the skills required for the transition are solidified, the latency-aged child is ready to engage the attainment of physical and mental skills of all kinds, such as prowess at individual and/or team sports, the ability to play musical instruments, and the elaboration of hobbies. All of these activities further the developmental process and lay the foundation for a rich intellectual and physical life in adolescence and beyond.

Latency falls within Piaget's stage of concrete operations. In essence, the latency-aged child is capable of formal learning because he or she can think rather than act, consider variables, similar and dissonant, and begin to understand time. Ancillary information and past experience can be brought into play as a more reality-centered viewpoint is formulated.

Erikson (1963) focused his brief consideration of latency on the child's ability to acquire useful skills. The desire to acquire knowledge of the tools of his or her culture and how to use them is called *industry*. The danger of not learning how to feel productive is that it results in feelings of inferiority. "Many a child's development is disrupted when family life has failed to prepare him for school life, or when school life fails to sustain the promises of earlier development" (p. 260).

PLAY IN CHILDHOOD

Play is an integral part of the life of children. Although it begins before and continues after latency, the forms and functions of play in childhood are presented here because in many ways this form of activity characterizes latency more than any other.

Occurring throughout childhood, indeed, throughout life, play occupies much of the young child's time. As one principal noted about his third graders, "When they're at recess, I can't stop them from playing." This pressure to play is an aspect of the important position which play occupies in the psychic life of the child, serving as a major vehicle for the engagement and mastery of developmental tasks.

The romanticized sense of play as random, carefree activity is far removed from its purposeful, psychically determined nature. As defined by Waelder (1932/1976) "play may now be characterized as a method of constantly working over and, as it were, assimilating piecemeal an experience which was too large to be assimilated instantly at one swoop" (pp. 217–218). In other words, because of the immaturity of their psychic apparatus, young children cannot quickly or easily integrate new experiences. As Waelder put it, "traumatic stimulation in childhood is the general rule" (p. 217). Instead, they repeat aspects of their inner world and actual events over and over again in an attempt at mastery. That is why an understanding of a child's play is so important clinically; it contains the major thoughts, feelings, and conflicts of the child expressed through actions and words which are comfortable and natural for the young patient.

This basic urge to repeat in an attempt at mastery, called the *repetition compulsion,* is observed throughout life in both normal and pathological circumstances. For example, the repetition compulsion is a basic characteristic of posttraumatic stress disorders. A second mechanism utilized in play is that of activity over passivity. Using this process, first observed in infancy, the child actively manipulates his or her play in an attempt to master an event which was experienced passively. For example, take the 4-year-old who receives a painful shot from the pediatrician and comes home and plays doctor, sticking a doll over and over again, making the doll "cry." This example illustrates why play is such an illuminating process for the child therapist; through it the child reveals that which is troubling him or her, making the conflicts accessible to the therapeutic process.

But play is not always an expression of the child's reaction to an actual event; it may also represent a wish or a fantasy. For example, caught in the midst of a divorce, a 7-year-old patient repeatedly played house and brought his father back into his life. In the playhouse, his mother and father loved each other and spent time with their children.

Building on Waelder's pioneering work, Lili Peller (1954) approached play developmentally, describing a topic, anxiety, and compensating fantasy for each developmental phase. During the first and second year of life, play originates in relationship to the body as the child paraphrases and magnifies various functions. Later, Mahler would describe this activity as "practicing." As the child uses toys and materials, such as sand or water, to substitute for body parts, he or she is concerned that the body is inadequate and in a compensatory manner fantasizes that it is a perfect instrument for the expression of wishes. Another variation of early play related to separation–individuation issues is the "peekaboo game."

Between the ages of 1 and 3, play primarily reflects the child's relationship with the omnipotent, omniscient preoedipal mother. Through countless repetitions, which often bore adults, the toddler does to toys and teddy bears what mother does to him or her. Play during these years is solitary or involves mother and other significant caretakers. For the most part, children do not play together at this age. Rather they play alongside each other in what has been called *parallel play.*

Play as most adults conceptualize it refers to the activities of Oedipal-aged and latency-aged children. Between the ages of 3 to 6, play is quite idiosyncratic because it is organized around the fantasies of the individual child. However, there is similarity in theme among children in this age group because they are dealing with the same dynamic issues: "Let's play house. I'll be the mommy. You be the daddy. You be the baby." For the first time, other children play distinct and separate roles in the play, which is elaborated spontaneously as it proceeds.

The basic anxiety is, "I am small and left out of adult pleasures and prerogatives"; the compensatory fantasy, "I am big and can do what adults do." This identification with adults lends a quality of triumph and naive invincibility to the play; for example, "I'm as strong as Wonder Woman" or "I can run faster than you, daddy."

. With the onset of latency, play changes dramatically because of a combination of maturational, social, and internal factors. Growth is steady and even, coordination is greatly enhanced. The newly acquired abilities to read, to count and write, and to relate independently to peers broadens the range of possibilities. Last, but not least, the internalization of the superego is reflected in the ubiquitousness of rules and punishment. No longer are games based on individual fantasies as they were during the Oedipal phase. In latency, they are learned from peers who in turn learned them from those who came before them; in other words, they are reflections of the culture.

According to Peller, the dynamics of latency play are focused on the fear of dealing with the anxiety related to facing the superego alone and the compensatory fantasy of being part of a group which shares the anxiety and follows rules to the letter. Whereas Oedipal play is focused on the future and the wish to grow up, latency play is organized around turning the clock back, getting another chance to start over, to do better, and to appease and please the superego.

Examples of latency-aged play are kickball and Monopoly. Kickball, a popular game on the playground which is similar to baseball, requires physical coordination and the ability to relate to teammates. Interlocking roles, such as pitcher, batter, and fielder, are required as are opponents. All aspects of the game are governed by rules and punishment—three strikes you're out, three outs and your side loses its turn. Willingness to tolerate frustration and control impulses is implicit. Monopoly requires the ability to read and a knowledge of mathematics as well as sophisticated concepts, such as saving, selling and buying, and trading. Once again, rules are everywhere. Take your turn; pass GO and collect $200; go directly to jail; do not pass GO; do not collect $200.

Although the form of play does not change significantly after latency—adolescents and adults continue to play baseball, checkers, and Monopoly—the reason why they play change dramatically, reflecting the major developmental preoccupations of each phase. For example, in midlife the normative anxiety about time limitation and personal death is momentarily mastered by the opportunity to conquer time through play.

In tennis there is always another game, another set, another match, the opportunity to reverse time and begin anew.

THE LITERATURE OF LATENCY

Another reflection of the qualitative developmental changes of latency is found in the literature of latency. Through universally loved fairy tales, movies, comics, and TV programs, the latency-aged child deals with the major developmental themes of the first decade of life.

The hero is often a child who has magical powers or associates with those who possess them in order to compensate for feelings of impotence in the mysterious adult world. Examples are Peter Pan, Alice (in Wonderland), and Dorothy in *The Wizard of Oz*. Aspects of narcissism and egocentricity are reflected in the absence of siblings. When brothers or sisters are present, they are often ugly and awful as in *Cinderella*. Sometimes animals or unusual characters represent various aspects of the self and others, as exemplified by Bambi and the dwarfs in *Snow White*.

The reflection of the superego is everywhere, sometimes almost literally as in *Pinocchio* where Jimminy Cricket sits on Pinocchio's shoulder and whispers advice and warnings in his ear; or the absence of vagueness in regard to right and wrong. Heroes are *very* good, such as Superman and Wonder Woman; villains, very bad, such as Captain Hook and the Wicked Witch of the West. Heroes use their superhuman powers in the service of good and justice and never deviate from the straight and narrow, at least until Superman used his X-ray vision in the movie version to see the color of Lois Lane's underwear.

Oedipal themes are everywhere. Take, for example, the competition between Snow White and the Wicked Queen—"Mirror, mirror on the wall, who is the fairest of them all?"—or the competition between Cinderella and her stepmother and stepsisters for the favor of the handsome prince. The wish to possess the Oedipal object is expressed but stripped of any signs of overt sexuality. Snow White can only be awakened from the sleeping spell put on her by the queen by a kiss from a handsome prince, but it is as pristine a peck as one can imagine. In Cinderella, the prince can only be won by the maiden whose foot "fits" the shoe placed upon it by the prince in his determined search to find his beloved. In both of these stories, the elaboration of Oedipal fantasies is strictly forbidden, swept under the rug into the unconscious by the superego with that greatest of generalities, "and they lived happily everafter."

By late latency and early adolescence the literature begins to reflect a new sophistication. The heroes are often real persons, such as Babe Ruth and Helen Keller, or children who use their intelligence and wit to challenge the intricacies and mysteries of the adult world, such as the Hardy Boys and Nancy Drew. Those who wish to explore this subject in more depth are referred to Bruno Bettleheim's (1976) book *The Uses of Enchantment: The Meaning and Importance of Fairy Tales.*

PREPARING FOR ADOLESCENCE

Latency is a time of separating from parents and entering the community, resolving the Oedipal conflict and internalizing the superego, developing peer relationships, and acquiring formal learning and hobbies. All of these positive developmental steps are not only important in their own right, but are also essential in creating a solid foundation, a reservoir of strength to help weather the psychological upheaval of adolescence which lies just ahead. Assessing the degree of mastery of these developmental tasks of latency will help the diagnostician determine the depth of adolescent pathology and the ability of patient and therapist to work together successfully.

CHAPTER 7

Adolescence (Ages 12–20)

Adolescence begins with a well-defined, maturational event, *puberty*, and ends in a more nebulous manner. Chronologically the end of adolescence is usually defined by the attainment of age 20, but mastery of the psychological tasks of adolescence continues well into young adulthood. This phase of development is usually subdivided into four parts: preadolescence (ages 11–13), early adolescence (ages 13–15), middle adolescence (ages 15–17) and late adolescence (ages 17–19).

PUBERTY

Puberty refers to the biological and psychological events which surround the first menstruation in the girl and the first ejaculation in the boy. These events signal the beginning of a process of profound physical change which renders the psychic organization of latency inadequate to the task of managing the physically and sexually mature body. In a simplified manner, adolescence may be defined as those years in which the mind develops the capacity to integrate these changes in relationship to self and to other (Erikson, 1956). Much of the material in this chapter is extracted from the classical text, *On Adolescence* by Peter Blos (1962). The reader is referred to this work as a starting point for obtaining a more thorough understanding of adolescent psychology.

The details of the growth spurt and sexual changes which characterize the pre- and postpubertal period are well known and will not be described here; however, the psychological responses to these events will be treated because of their clinical relevance. Many children are referred for evaluation at this time either because of their reaction to puberty or the timing of its onset (normally between ages 12 and 14, earlier in girls than in boys).

If the years prior to adolescence have been characterized by problematic development, puberty may precipitate the onset of significant symptomatology. This may occur even in those individuals who had undergone "successful" psychotherapy or analysis during the Oedipal or latency years; because adolescence requires a major reworking of *all* aspects of earlier development, in the process exposing and amplifying weaknesses.

Those children who begin puberty either very early or very late are particularly vulnerable because they are so out of step physically and psychologically with their peers. An example would be the 17-year-old prepubertal male who was referred because of suicidal ideation after a girl laughed at him when he asked her to the junior prom. A careful evaluation revealed that he was not significantly impaired psychologically but was desperately unhappy because he was "like a baby in high school." The spontaneous onset of puberty 11 months later and 2 years of psychotherapy led to a tumultuous, but successful leap into late adolescence!

THE DEVELOPMENTAL TASKS OF ADOLESCENCE

Accepting the Physically and Sexually Mature Body

The physical transition from an immature to a mature body takes several years. Because body growth is uneven and uncontrollable, it is accompanied, even in the most beautiful girl or handsome boy, with periodic losses in self-esteem and injured narcissism. As the adolescent compares his or her body with that of his peers and adults, real or imagined differences are magnified and distorted. Legs, arms, and noses are too long; pimples too gross and obvious; and in private thought or conversation with best friends, breasts and penises are too small—or too big.

Because others in the peer group are experiencing the same doubts, some individuals use cruel comments about another's body in order to externalize their own pain. One 13-year-old girl was nearly hysterical as she told me how a boy in her class had teased her about her breasts in front of his friends. "Pretty soon you're going to need bushel baskets to carry them around," he said.

The slowly growing, comfortable body of latency is gone, replaced by one of great, and potentially disastrous, unpredictability. In boys, spontaneous erections may occur at any time, most likely when called upon to stand up in front of others in class or in the shower after physical education. In girls, the menstrual cycle is not very regular at first; consequently, one must be constantly on guard against mortifying spots of "blood." Wet dreams occur with increasing regularity, announcing to the mother that her son is, as one boy put it, "either masturbating or wetting the bed. I don't want her to know anything about what's happening to me."

As these changes are accepted and integrated, the body once again becomes a consistent source of pride and pleasure. Hours are spent in early adolescence examining body parts, primping in private or in front of the mirror, and combing and recombing the hair. Tight clothes are used to display the body to others. There is nothing quite so grand as the 15- or 16-year-old proudly displaying his or her body for all to admire.

Feelings of doubt and desires to exhibit are often in conflict with each other. One 14-year-old girl sat across from me alternately slumping in her chair, with her arms folded across her chest, and thrusting out her breasts, with no apparent awareness of what she was doing.

All these ideas are extremely important for clinicians because insensitivity to the adolescent's feelings about his or her body can disrupt or destroy a therapeutic relationship. Comments, even positive ones, about clothing, grooming, or the body itself, should be avoided until a relationship is well established. Even then, anything to do with the body must be approached with tact, sensitivity, and emotional neutrality.

Separating Physically and Psychologically from Parents

Referring to Margaret Mahler's separation–individuation theory, Peter Blos (1967) called adolescence the time of the "second individuation." Just as the infant must separate and individuate from the mother, so must the adolescent initiate the process of physical and psychological separation from parents and home which will allow him or her to function as an autonomous, independent young adult. The attainment of physical and cognitive maturity makes it possible for the adolescent to approach self-sufficiency; the onset of sexual maturity makes it imperative that he or she direct sexual feelings outside the family. At the beginning of this transition phase, the child is dependent on his or her family of origin and is sexually immature; at the end of it, the young adult is independent and sexually active, ready to establish a family of procreation. As we shall see in our discussion of young adulthood, the processes of psychological separation and sexual identity formation are by no means complete at the end of adolescence; they continue to be elaborated throughout the young adult years and beyond.

Knowledge of the second individuation will help the clinician understand and successfully treat many adolescent patients, whether they present with homesickness on going to camp, difficulty in making friends or dating, or an inability to leave home for college.

Clinical example: L. had a very unhappy adolescence because she was unable to gain acceptance in her peer group and could not find a boyfriend. These problems had their roots in the first individuation (an exaggerated dependence on her mother) and the Oedipal phase (a psychologically seductive relationship with her father). After a particularly cruel rejection by a group of girlfriends in tenth grade, L. turned her attention and affections toward a girl 3 years her junior. This sublimated homosexual relationship and a continuing close relationship with both parents sustained L. through the social and sexual isolation of the last 2 years of high school. Psychotherapy initiated during her senior year was prematurely interrupted by L.'s decision to "go for broke" and matriculate to a college far from home. There she spent a miserable, isolated year. Transfer to a college in her hometown and the reestablishment of contact with the best friend, parents, and therapist provided symptomatic relief and the opportunity to work in depth on the unresolved aspects of the first and second individuation.

Accepting Sexual Maturation and Establishing an Active Sexual Life

The developmental line of sexual identity is greatly expanded in adolescence by the need to accept the sexually mature body and to begin to establish an active sexual life. The course along this developmental line may be divided into three phases which correspond to the generally recognized subdivisions of early, middle, and late adolescence. In pre- and early adolescence, the tasks are to accept the sexually mature body; particularly, the growth of underarm and pubic hair and the enlargement of the genitals and breasts; and to explore through masturbation new sexual functions, such as increased vaginal lubrication and ejaculation. Building on this still shaky foundation, the middle adolescent makes tentative steps toward the opposite sex, but handles most sexual feelings through fantasy and masturbation rather than actual involvement with others. By late adolescence, most individuals are psychologically prepared for an active sexual life which includes intercourse.

This normative timetable will help the clinician place adolescent patients on this developmental line and define sexual issues which need to be explored in therapy. Particular emphasis should be placed upon the content of sexual fantasies, especially masturbatory ones, which are the intrapsychic indicators of how well the adolescent is separating his or her sexuality from parents, and redirecting them toward appropriate, non-incestuous partners.

The absence of progression along this line (in the presence of sexual maturity) often indicates neurotic inhibition. However, early sexual experience is not an indicator of rapid developmental progression; it, too, often suggests the presence of pathology, which is related to problems with impulse control and/or lack of parental involvement in limit setting. Understanding adolescent sexual functioning is difficult at best but almost impossible without a thorough understanding of the patient's previous experience along the developmental line of sexual identity and a detailed knowledge of current fantasy life and activity.

Preparing to Work

When a 5-year-old says he or she wants to be an astronaut or a garbage collector, adults smile; but when an adolescent expresses preferences, everyone listens seriously. In a sense, it is ironic that adolescents are forced to make major decisions about work and career (by exclusion or choice) which will affect the rest of their lives at a time when they are so preoccupied with physical, sexual, and social interests. In some countries, such as Britain and China, where only 1% to 2% of the population are allowed to go on to college on the basis of evaluations of their potential which are made in adolescence, future choice is severely limited. In countries, such as the United States, the options for future education and work and professional advancement remain open indefinitely; hence, adolescent decisions about career choice are less momentous.

Preparing for an adult career during adolescence is dependent on numerous ego strengths and superego and ego ideal functions, such as the ability to delay gratification, channel impulses, sublimate, develop cognitive capacities and motor skills, visualize the future, and conceptualize oneself as an adult at work rather than a child at play.

The degree to which work during adolescence stimulates or impedes the expansion of developmental potential varies enormously from individual to individual. For some, particularly those who are planning to enter a trade or non-college related work, experience gained on the job during the adolescent years may be highly valuable and gratifying. For

others, regardless of whether or not their future plans require higher
education, spending time working during adolescence may impede the
development of social, emotional, and sexual skills and attitudes which
will be highly useful in the adult workplace.

IDENTITY VERSUS ROLE CONFUSION

Erikson (1963) described adolescence as a time of struggle over
identity.

> The growing and developing youths, faced with this psychological revolution
> within them, and with tangible adult tasks ahead of the are now primarily
> concerned with what they appear to be in the eyes of others as compared with
> what they feel they are and with the question of how to connect the roles and
> skills cultivated earlier with the occupational prototypes of the day. (p. 261)

If the adolescent is unable to master the developmental tasks of
the phase, role confusion results—confusion over individuality, sexuality,
and a place in the adult world.

REACTIONS TO PUBERTY

Because of an outpouring of growth and sexual hormones, the comfortable balance between mind and body which existed in latency is
shattered. Suddenly the impulses are stronger than the capacities of the
ego and superego to regulate and control them. This imbalance is similar
in nature to that which existed between the ages of 1 to 3 and caused the
developmental disturbances of the toddler.

Regression in the form of silliness and immature and unpredictable
behavior is a common normative response as is the shift from openness
to secretiveness. At home, the secretiveness is manifested by increased
demands for privacy and refusal to share information about activities
(Blos, 1970). Parents who do not understand the developmental purpose
of this phenomenon will be wounded and angry. Clinicians who expect
openness and consistent cooperation will experience similar feelings. At
school and in the peer group the secretiveness is reflected in the formation of secret clubs, cliques, and "best" friendships in which sexual information (and misinformation) is shared and pooled.

Clothing suddenly takes on an exaggerated importance. It is used to
draw attention to, or away from, the new sexualized body, as evidence of
acceptance by a clique or club, and as an indicator of autonomy and
independence from parents. Hairstyles, makeup, and other body adorn-

ments serve similar functions. By allowing the adolescent to freely choose clothing and hairstyles—within broadly set limits—the understanding parent supports the drive toward autonomy and healthy sexuality.

Clinicians look at the adolescent's clothing, hairstyle, and adornments as a potential source of insight into his or her dynamics. One 13-year-old male regularly dressed in steel-tipped shoes, ripped jeans, and a tee shirt proclaiming "Hitler's Triumphant Tour Across Europe." This dress and his unsmiling countenance were meant to intimidate and disgust peers and adults alike, a goal that was easily accomplished. The defensive function of such a presentation, covering feelings of rage and unacceptability because of rejection by both natural and adoptive parents, gradually became apparent and were eventually interpreted to the patient. Subsequent modification of appearance and simultaneous work on relationships with parents and on sexuality eventually produced in this adolescent increased social acceptance, sexual involvement with girlfriends, and greater self-confidence.

PEER RELATIONSHIPS AND FRIENDSHIPS

From the latency period onward, friendships play a central role in human experience as they are shaped by the mutual needs to engage and resolve phase-specific developmental tasks. In early adolescence, in particular, developmental pressures may strain the capacity for friendships because the sexual and aggressive drives are temporarily so much stronger than the abilities of the ego and superego to contain them. This can lead to breakdowns in aim inhibition as observed in both homosexual and heterosexual experimentation between peers. However, at no other point in the life cycle do friendships play such a prominent role in the developmental process, thereby facilitating the engagement and resolution of such critical developmental tasks as psychological separation from parents and the beginning integration of adult attitudes toward work, play, and sexuality.

Girls who begin their maturation spurt 1 to 2 years before boys are quite often stronger and taller. These "young Amazons" often belittle their male peers and are attracted to older boys. Within the same-sex peer group, they are often exceedingly cruel to each other, shifting loyalties on a day-to-day basis and openly attacking competitors and enemies. The reasons for such behavior are multiple and include the displacement of ambivalent feelings about the parents, insecurity about the physical and sexual changes which are occurring, and the weakening of superego controls. Because early adolescent girls are physically developed and can present a pseudomature posture, they sometimes rush toward mid- and late-adolescent social and sexual behavior for which they are unprepared psychologically. Parental limits are extremely important in preventing inappropriate involvements. Therapists need to understand that despite their physically and socially mature presentation, early adolescent girls, like their male counterparts, are still dealing with the developmental tasks of psychologically separating from parents and understanding and accepting the sexually mature body. As a consequence, they are not ready for intense relationships.

Pre- and early adolescent boys are quite threatened by these young Amazons and cover their emerging sexual feelings and fears with bravado, boasting, and even physical attacks. They maintain, for the most part, that latency attitude of "hating" girls and are most comfortable in same-sex peer groups. Group activities, such as Boy Scouts, camping, and organized sports, help the boy to separate from his parents and channel sexual and aggressive energies within a structured framework.

For both sexes, but particularly for boys because of their physical immaturity in comparison to girls and their tendency to manage their sexual feelings in same-sex peer groups, pre- and early adolescence is a time of "normal" homosexual experimentation. Both sexes compare physical changes and engage in mutual masturbation. The basic purpose of such activity is to gain reassurance about the momentous physical and sexual changes which are occurring. In those individuals whose sexual orientation is basically heterosexual, such behavior ceases as the changes in the body are psychologically integrated and gradually replaced by involvement with the opposite sex.

Clinicians need to utilize this information and a detailed knowledge of the individual's past experience along the developmental line of sexual identity in order to assess the normality or pathology of sexual behavior in pre- and early adolescence, recognizing that sexual orientation remains open to influence from the sexual experiences of mid- and late adolescence and young adulthood, and is not "fixed" in adolescence.

The developmental line leading to an adult homosexual orientation will not be considered in this discussion because there is little agreement (and in my opinion, insufficient knowledge) about the developmental processes which result in an adult homosexual orientation. Also, despite the position statement by the American Psychiatric Association that homosexuality is not a pathological entity, considerable controversy remains about the normality or pathology of adult homosexuality.

THE RELATIONSHIP BETWEEN ADOLESCENTS
AND THEIR PARENTS

Pre- and early adolescence brings an uncomfortable change in the relationship between parent and child. Gone is the easy openness, affability, and mutual admiration of late latency. In its stead are avoidance, secretiveness, and public embarrassment. ("Mom, please drop me off a block from school. I don't want my friends to see us together!") on the part of the adolescent, and bewilderment, sadness, and anger on the part of parents. The degree to which these attitudes are present varies. Often they alternate with the long-established closeness and mutuality which form the basis of the normal relationship between parent and child at all points in the life cycle, including adolescence.

The dynamic forces driving the child are multiple, relating to both current and past developmental themes. In the present, the powerful hormonally driven sexuality affects all relationships, including those with parents. What was a comfortable, easily managed emotional interaction just a few months ago is suddenly contaminated by an unwelcome sexual component. Hugs and kisses, indeed any form of contact with the mother or the father's body, may produce feelings of discomfort and stimulate conscious or unconscious sexual feelings and fantasies. The body can no longer be counted on to respond to closeness in predictable ways since a fleeting touch or extended hug may produce an erect penis or nipples. Bedroom and bathroom doors are suddenly locked tight to distance parents from the pubescent body.

At an unconscious level, the repression of the Oedipal complex, maintained with relative ease during latency, is now threatened by the power of the hormonally driven fantasies, raising the prospect of the return to consciousness of blatant sexual fantasies about the parents. But unlike the Oedipal-aged child, the early adolescent is capable of having intercourse. The possibility that the incest barrier may be breached by the sexual maturity of the adolescent forces a reworking and further abandonment of Oedipal fantasies and wishes. As we shall see in our discussion of adult development, the Oedipal complex is never completely "resolved" or abandoned; rather it is altered and transformed by developmental pressures throughout the life course.

Aspects of this conflict are often observed in relationship to the adolescent's bedroom. Signs on the door, such as "Parents—Keep Out!" although unnerving, underline one of the developmental processes taking place. Insistence on wild decor, suggestive posters, and the absence of neatness and cleanliness are all indicators of the intense need to create the semblance of independence from parental space and values, while remaining in their secure, protective midst. Wise parents will tolerate all but the most outlandish and extreme remodeling efforts, recognizing the benign aspects of such rebellion and standoffishness. When confined to the home, such behavior, although not conducive to parental peace and equanimity, facilitates the developmental process and is self-limiting. One father, objecting to the presence of "pictures of Bruce Springsteen's crotch all over my daughter's bedroom walls," was mildly placated by the comment that they were, after all, only pictures. His daughter was practicing a form of safe adolescent sex—fantasy! He was also reassured by the recognition that his daughter's behavior and surly attitude seemed reserved for him and his wife. Neighbors, friends, and teachers still spoke of her in glowing terms, indicating the presence of judgment and responsible behavior in the midst of developmental regression and turmoil.

Although the Oedipal component to adolescent sexuality may be obvious to the clinician, it may not be to the patient. Consequently, considerable care must be taken when interpreting aspects of sexual fantasies and behavior. For example, a 14-year-old neurotic boy, in therapy for over a year, revealed with embarrassment, but without understanding, that he regularly masturbated on his parents' bed. Lying face down on his mother's side, he simulated the motions of intercourse, trying hard to ejaculate on the toilet paper which was strategically placed beneath his penis. Eventually, the connection between his masturbation and his sexual wishes for his mother were interpreted, leading to a change in masturbatory activity and greater intrapsychic separation from the mother.

A second major theme from the infantile past which must be reworked at this time is the unconscious relationship with the preoedipal mother (Brunswick, 1940), the omnipotent, omniscient progenitor of the first few years of life. Both boys and girls must come to see mother in a less potent, more imperfect light, gradually assuming more and more of her power for themselves. Both sexes tend to have a more conflictual relationship with the mother than with the father as they ward off and work through the dependent wishes for fusion, not unlike the toddler did many years before. Then as now, the father, always seen in a more rational, balanced light, is available to modulate and moderate, serving as a go-between for both the mother and the child. Just as the toddler required the consistent presence of the parents in order to work through aspects of the first individuation, so does the adolescent need regular contact with parents in order to safely master the developmental tasks just described. The parental role is a mixture of consistent caring and the exercise of mature judgment and limit setting, while gradually allowing the adolescent increased freedom and responsibility.

Probably at no point in the life cycle is the relationship between child and adult development more apparent than in the interaction between adolescent and young adult and middle-aged parent. Before the advent of a comprehensive developmental theory of adulthood, parents were assumed to be finished products, pillars of stability attempting to contain the adolescent tempest. Now we understand that parental reaction to adolescent children is strongly influenced by developmental conflict in the parent as well. Gerald Pearson first introduced this idea of "the conflict of generations" in 1955 and Robert Nemiroff and I subsequently elaborated it (Colarusso & Nemiroff, 1981). We will consider the parental issues in detail in Chapters Ten and Eleven on young and middle adulthood.

Problems in the adolescent–parent relationship are a frequent reason for referral and an issue of critical importance to both adolescent and adult patients. Once again, a knowledge of the developmental processes at work will help the clinician formulate a diagnosis and treatment plan and increase the chances that both adolescent and parent will be understood.

THE SUPEREGO AND THE EGO IDEAL

The Superego

The superego which was so effective in comfortably controlling fantasy and behavior in late latency is less so in early adolescence because of an increase in the power of the impulses and the psychological withdrawal from parents and their representations in the superego (Loewald, 1979). Thus, during this interval in early adolescence, when the superego is being restructured to include the new capability for sexual and aggressive expression, a necessary developmental step, controls on behavior are less reliable and the adolescent is highly vulnerable to influences to act in inappropriate ways, particularly when that pressure comes from peers. Even in stable individuals there may be an increase in lying, cheating, and stealing.

Larry was a 13-year-old boy in treatment for fears and phobias. His past history was characterized by restriction and inhibition, not impulsivity. One day he described a completely uncharacteristic experience for him. At a friend's suggestion, the boys decided to throw eggs at passing cars. When the police showed up, the boys ran, jumping over back fences in their successful avoidance of their pursuers.

The risk of acting out during this period of transition may be diminished by close parental involvement and supervision and careful monitoring of the peer group. Even as the adolescent is withdrawing from parental influences and restrictions in both the real and intrapsychic worlds, he or she tends to draw parents into conflicts over controls, thus ensuring some external restraint.

Therapists must walk a fine line, filled with anxiety and concern, as they observe and facilitate the process of superego restructuring which is often accompanied by dangerous behavior. For example, one late adolescent would cross the border into Mexico every weekend with his friends to drink and carouse. Despite my pleas for caution and restraint, particularly in regard to carrying marijuana into a Third World country, he continued this behavior for months, aware of the danger but certain that "They'll never get me. I'm too lucky." Fortunately, they never did.

The healthy adolescent uses fantasy, autoerotic activities, and the reengagement of latency-aged activities to minimize the tendency toward action. One girl reorganized her stamp collection. Another began a library with her best friend, while a boy became reinvested in baseball cards.

The Ego Ideal

Peter Blos (1974) suggested that the adolescent developmental process results in the formation of a new psychic structure, the ego ideal. In essence, the ego ideal is that part of the personality which contains the individual's highest future expectations of himself or herself. The ego ideal is regarded as a part of the superego in the view of some clinicians. Blos emphasized the need for an adolescent revision and expansion of the superego to encompass the emerging adult aspirations for sex, intimacy, and work achievement.

In order for this to occur, the infantile idealization of the parents and their expectations for their "child" which are already internalized in the superego must be diminished and eventually replaced by a new set of standards which reflect the adolescent's sexual and mental maturity, ambitions, and goals and the influence of nonincestuous friends, lovers, and mentors. The process of "deidealization" begins in early adolescence when these loving, idealized feelings are transferred from the parents to a best friend who acquires some of the emotional significance of the progenitors. Thus, these friendships are transitional, facilitating the movement from dependent child to autonomous adult.

The relationship with the best friend is almost palpable, so intense is the emotional investment. Through identification, certain qualities of the friend are internalized and then, having served its developmental purpose, the relationship diminishes in significance or disappears completely, often to be replaced by another of similar intensity and duration. These seemingly homosexual attachments are phase-appropriate precursors of the heterosexual crushes and infatuations which represent the next step in the progression toward adult sexuality.

THE TRANSITION TO
HETEROSEXUALITY—FALLING IN LOVE

During middle adolescence, following the acceptance of the physically and sexually mature body and the formation of the ego ideal, there is a gradual turn toward heterosexuality. These early efforts to engage the opposite sex are both thrilling and frightening. When one's affections are returned, the result, immortalized in song and verse, is the experience of falling in love, more properly called adolescent infatuation. A necessary prerequisite to, but quite different from mature, adult love, infatuation furthers developmental progress by loosening the intrapsychic ties to the Oedipal objects and providing experience with loving and sexual feelings in a nonincestuous relationship. But in a sense, the adolescent falls in love with the idealized parent of childhood, characteristics of whom are projected onto the boyfriend or girlfriend. This necessary developmental step in the process of intrapsychic separation from the parents makes it difficult to see the new loved one in a realistic light. This explains why the sense of disillusionment in the boyfriend or girlfriend is so strong when the projected idealization is withdrawn.

In addition, adolescent infatuations help resolve homosexual and bisexual trends by providing a repository for feminine traits in the male and masculine traits in the female. For example, when a girl loves and is loved in return, she can project her masculine interests onto her boyfriend, enjoying them in him while feeling feminine and loved. The same thing in reverse is true for the boy. When sexual involvement is part of the relationship, passive and active trends may be expressed and experimented with within a comfortable setting. This mutual identification is basic to the infatuation and is refined with each succeeding relationship. In marriage, it becomes an essential mechanism for the more definitive resolution of bisexual trends and the elaboration of parental identity.

Because of the tenuous nature of these relationships, there is a great fear of rejection, often actualized, and the inevitable experience of narcissistic injury. The ability to engage in a number of infatuations is a sign of strength and resilience, since despite the pain involved when they end, each relationship leads to greater separation and individuation. Therapists should be concerned about the absence of attempts at involvement, often indicating neurotic inhibition, or the rush into an intense relationship which continues throughout middle and late adolescence, sometimes leading to marriage. Both experiences tend to be defensive, protecting the individual from the loneliness, uncertainty, and rejection which are inevitable aspects of adolescent infatuation.

Healthy adolescents have many sources of narcissistic gratification and supply to cushion the pain of loneliness and rejection and fill the time between infatuations. Elaboration of latency-aged interests, a focus on intellectual tasks and athletics, and the pursuit of such hobbies as auto mechanics or collecting all provide nonsexualized pleasure and facilitate sublimation and the acquisition of valuable skills and abilities which will serve the adolescent well into adulthood.

SEXUAL IDENTITY IN LATE ADOLESCENCE

By late adolescence, most individuals have accepted the body as a sexual instrument, partially replaced the parents as primary love objects, and begun an active sexual life. For others, work on these themes continues into young adulthood. Before the advent of an organized theory of adulthood, it was postulated that the developmental line of sexual identity ended with late adolescence, with all of the capabilities for mature, adult sexuality firmly in place. Now it is recognized that adolescent sexuality is one phase of a lifelong process of sexual evolution. In Chapter Ten we will focus on the young adult developmental themes of intimacy, mature love, and parenthood, all of which build upon adolescent experience and integration.

COGNITIVE DEVELOPMENT

According to Piaget (1954), adolescence is the phase of development in which thinking reaches its highest level, what he called *formal operational thinking*. As we shall see in the chapters on adulthood, many other researchers have suggested that cognitive development continues well beyond adolescence, producing forms of thought that are more advanced than formal operations.

The adolescent is capable of greater degrees of abstraction. He or she can test assumptions and construct theories without as much reference to the concrete world. In addition, as every parent and therapist knows, adolescents develop the capacity to critically assess and logically evaluate ideas, both their own and others (Anthony, 1982). In late adolescence, in particular, the ability to abstract and the transformation of the superego and the ego ideal produce the idealism and expectation for societal change which are so characteristic of these years.

The nature of adolescent thought produces major changes in the therapeutic process. Play becomes a peripheral activity, eventually disappearing completely, and is replaced by "play" with thoughts, fantasies, and ideas. Insights and interpretations—of patient's *and* therapist's words and behavior—come from the adolescent as well as the adult. However, the ability to exercise mature judgment and use the insights acquired in therapy may remain limited because of an inability to control impulses and the depth of pathology present.

CHAPTER 8

A Historical Overview and General Principles of Adult Development

ANCIENT REFERENCES

The concept of the life cycle and adult development is nearly as old as recorded history. For instance, Solon (ca. 630–560 B.C.), the ancient Greek philosopher and poet, described six periods of adulthood and assigned developmental tasks to each, such as developing one's capabilities to the fullest and increasing in virtue. Shortly thereafter, Confucius (551–479 B.C.) described life experience in terms of age-related issues, such as setting one's heart to learning at 15 years of age, planting one's feet firmly on the ground at 30, knowing the biddings of heaven at 50, and following the dictates of the heart at 60. This idea of a continuous developmental process and change was eventually expressed in the lifelong Confucian quest for self-realization. Similar notions are embedded in Western thought, in the Talmudic prescription for the successive stages of maturation in the faith, and in the Christian quest for satisfaction and salvation, which addresses all major adult developmental themes.

Other references to the nature of developmental change throughout life are ubiquitous in classical and in contemporary literature. Not surprisingly, one of the most famous references is from that most intuitive of developmental observers, William Shakespeare:

> And one man in his time plays many parts,
> His acts being seven ages. At first the infant,
> Mewling and puking in the nurse's arms.

Then the whining schoolboy, with his satchel
And shining morning face, creeping like snail
Unwilling to school. And then the lover,
Sighing like furnace, with a woeful ballad
Made to his mistress' eyebrow. Then a soldier,
Full of strange oaths and bearded like the pard,
Jealous in honor, sudden and quick in quarrel,
Seeking the bubble reputation
Even in the cannon's mouth. And then the justice,
In fair round belly with good capon lined,
With eyes severe and beard of formal cut,
Full of wise saws and modern instances,
And so he plays his part. The sixth age shifts
Into the lean and slippered Pantaloon
With spectacles on nose and pouch on side,
His youthful hose, well saved, a world too wide
For his shrunk shank, and his big manly voice,
Turning again toward childish treble, pipes
And whistles in his sound. Last scene of all
That ends this strange eventful history,
Is second childishness and mere oblivion,
Sans teeth, sans eyes, sans taste, everything.
—*As You Like It*, II, vii

For a more detailed discussion of the ancient and more contemporary history of adult development, the reader is referred to Chapters 1 through 3 in *Adult Development* (Colarusso & Nemiroff, 1981), from which this brief historical overview is taken.

THE PIONEER DEVELOPMENTALISTS

The foundations of the current scientific interest in adult development are built upon the writings of four men, three psychiatrists and psychoanalysts, and one anthropologist. These contemporaries all made their major contributions in the first half of the twentieth century.

Arnold Van Gennep (1873–1957)

Arnold Van Gennep (1873–1957) was an anthropologist. In 1908 he published *The Rites of Passage* (Van Gennep, 1960), a monograph which studied cross culturally the manner in which individuals and societies mark and manage transitions from one phase of development to another. His work underscored the universality and dynamic nature of developmental processes while at the same time recognizing the enormous impact of cultural influence.

Sigmund Freud (1856–1939)

Although independently created, Freud's and Van Gennep's developmental hypotheses were published within three years of each other. In *The Three Essays on the Theory of Sexuality* (1905), Freud described the nature of the basic interactions between organism and environment which underlie all developmental processes. As maturationally determined potentials interact with environmental influences and stimulation, a predictable series of transformations and sequences occur (Abrams, 1978). Spitz's definition of development, often referred to in this book, is clearly based on these ideas of Freud. In addition, Freud introduced the concept of developmental stages and divided childhood into five parts. Although our current knowledge goes far beyond Freud's original conceptions, we still use his terms, *oral, anal, Oedipal, latency,* and *adolescence,* to describe development in childhood. Unfortunately, Freud did not apply his formulations to adulthood, a lapse which impeded for decades the emergence of a comprehensive developmental theory of adulthood.

Carl Gustav Jung (1875–1961)

Jung (1933) was one of the first researchers to suggest that the personality continued to evolve and change in adulthood. In this sense, as well as others, he went beyond Freud and forged his own theory. Recognizing the importance of biological retrogression and aging for psychic development in adulthood, Jung wrote intensively about midlife, which he called the "noon" of life. His notion that men become more aware of their feminine tendencies and women more in touch with their masculine strivings in midlife foreshadowed and stimulated the cross-cultural studies of David Gutmann (1971) on the same subject. Jung's balanced approach to the influence of child and adult experience is also contained in the archetypes "Puer" or Young and "Senes" or Old. These are the elemental unconscious images from the long history of human experience. Jung suggested that these primitive representations of young and old have an effect on attitudes toward aging and are modified by individual experience.

Erik H. Erikson (b. 1902)

Erikson's two greatest contributions to developmental theory are the division of the entire life cycle, not just childhood, into eight equally important stages and the description of a major dynamic polarity for each. The wide acceptance of his theories popularized the idea that development is lifelong, rather than ending with adolescence, and strongly influenced all contemporary adult developmental theoreticians. A child psychoanalyst who focused on the impact of social and cultural influences on the development of mental processes, Erikson underscored the importance of normative conflict for developmental progression. His well-known polarities of Intimacy versus Isolation (young adulthood), Generativity versus Stagnation (adulthood), and Ego Integrity versus Despair (late adulthood) were among the first delineations of adult developmental tasks and challenges. These ideas, like those for childhood which have already been described, were introduced in *Childhood and Society* (1963), a work undoubtedly familiar to most readers from their college courses or graduate studies. Erikson also explained how various cultures tailor childrearing practices to produce an adult personality structure which ensures their propagation and survival.

CONTEMPORARY ADULT DEVELOPMENTALISTS

Although a complex theory of child development has existed for decades, a comprehensive theory of adult development is just beginning to emerge. Stevens-Long (1979) suggested that the study of childhood preceded the study of adulthood because of economic, social, and psychological issues; particularly the spread of compulsory education and Freud's discovery of the influence of childhood experience on adult psychopathology. The more recent shift of interest to the adult years may be due to similar economic and social factors, particularly the increase in the life span by approximately 30 years during this century. The study of the second half of life is increasingly relevant and important if society is to understand and accommodate the rapidly growing numbers of older individuals.

For whatever reasons, the last 20 years have seen the emergence of adult development as a recognized field of study, increasingly included in graduate and postgraduate curricula. In this section on contemporary adult developmentalists, I will summarize the work of some of the better known researchers and suggest areas of study for the interested reader.

Daniel Levinson

Daniel Levinson and his associates have conducted systematic studies of adulthood and have published their results in *Seasons of a Man's Life* (Levinson, Darrow, & Klein, 1978). In their work, the life cycle is divided into 20-year intervals called *eras:* preadulthood, 0–20; early adulthood, 20–40; middle adulthood, 40–60; late adulthood, 60–80; and late late adulthood, 80 and beyond. Throughout life each individual constructs a series of evolving *life structures,* the underlying design for living at any given time, a pattern of the self in the world. When these life structures no longer meet the developmental demands of the time, they are revised intraphysically, producing periods of transition. Thus, each era consists of alternating intervals of stable structure and transition. For example, Levinson *et al.* defined three major intervals of transition for men between childhood and young adulthood, young and middle adulthood, and middle and late adulthood.

This body of theory, which evolved from the intensive study of relatively small numbers of men, has considerable clinical application, both in the understanding of midlife transition and midlife crisis (subjects which will be considered in Chapter Eleven, Middle Adulthood), and in the enhancement of the clinician's ability to identify salient themes behind adult symptoms.

George Vaillant

One of the few longitudinal studies of development is the Grant Study, which was begun at Harvard in 1939 when 268 male undergraduates were selected to be followed periodically with the use of interviews and questionnaires. Some of the findings of this ongoing study were reported by Vaillant in *Adaptation To Life* (1977) and more recently in an article in the *American Journal of Psychiatry* (1990). The findings confirm the basic developmental notions that life is lived most fully and successfully by those who engage the major developmental issues and themes of each successive phase of life, struggle with them, "master" them, and then move on to the next set of challenges. Examples would be developing a sexual life and intimacy during young adulthood and generativity during middle adulthood.

Focusing on mechanisms of defense, Vaillant discovered that there is a shift in usage, from a greater reliance on "immature" ones (acting out, hypochondriasis, and projection, among others) to the more frequent use of "mature" ones (suppression, altruism, sublimation, anticipation, and humor). This was one of the first studies to confirm the normative evolution of psychic structure in adulthood, undermining the idea that mental structures were relatively fixed and rigid at the end of adolescence.

Calvin A. Colarusso and Robert A. Nemiroff

In the late 1970s, Robert Nemiroff and I began to focus our attention on adult development. This interest grew out of the recognition that there was no body of developmental theory for the adult years as there was for childhood, and a desire to understand the effect of experiences beyond childhood on the symptomatology of our patients. Drawing primarily on our experience as practicing psychiatrists and psychoanalysts, we published in 1981 *Adult Development: A New Dimension in Psychodynamic Theory and Practice*. This volume was focused on an elaboration and codification of normal adult experience and the use of these concepts in the diagnosis and treatment of adults. Then, in *The Race against Time: Psychotherapy and Psychoanalysis in the Second Half of Life* (Nemiroff & Colarusso, 1985), we and several colleagues addressed the treatment of older patients, demonstrating the usefulness of dynamic treatment for patients from the ages of 40 through 80. This book was followed by the edited volume, *New Dimensions in Adult Development* (Nemiroff & Colarusso, 1990), a multidisciplinary effort, which presented the latest thinking in this rapidly expanding discipline, of over 20 leading scholars and clinicians who addressed a wide variety of subjects.

Bernice Neugarten and the Chicago School of Human Development

Through the study of large numbers of adults in nonclinical settings, Neugarten and her colleagues (1964; 1975; 1979) have contributed much to our understanding of individuals in middle and late adulthood. This included the increased awareness of aging and the personalization of death, expressed in body monitoring and a tendency to view time in terms of time-left-to-live rather than time-since-birth. Members of the middle generation normally develop a sense of competence unrealized earlier in life and have a unique perspective on the younger and older generations. As they grow older, they become more introspective, developing an increased "interiority," which culminates in late adulthood in the life review (Butler, 1963), a detailed appraisal of one's life as it nears an end.

Stimulated by these efforts and the work of many other individuals, the field of adult development has become recognized as a separate discipline, of interest to anthropologists, sociologists, historians, and philosophers, as well as clinicians. Among the many articles and books which have been published recently, the reader may find particular value in the revised and expanded versions of *The Course of Life* (1981), edited by Stanley Greenspan and George Pollock; *Normality and the Life Cycle* (1984), edited by Daniel Offer and Melvin Sabshin; *The Middle Years* (1989), edited by John M. Oldham and Robert Liebert; and *New Techniques in the Psychotherapy of Older Patients* (1991), edited by Wayne Myers.

HYPOTHESES ON THE NATURE OF
ADULT DEVELOPMENT

In an attempt to delineate aspects of the basic nature of adult development, Nemiroff and I (Colarusso & Nemiroff, 1981) formulated seven hypotheses. Although having gained considerable acceptance since they were first proposed over a decade ago, some hypotheses are still considered controversial. They are discussed here, at the beginning of the section on adulthood, to form a conceptual bridge to the material just presented on child development and to delineate areas of agreement and disagreement.

Hypothesis I: "The Nature of the Developmental Process is Basically the Same in the Adult as in the Child" (Colarusso & Nemiroff, 1981, p. 61). By that we meant, using Spitz's definition of development as a basis of our idea, that the adult personality, like that of the child, is continually shaped by biological, intrapsychic, and environmental influences. This idea contradicted the commonly held notion, as exemplified by the following Eissler quote (1975), that the adult is relatively free from biological and environmental influences:

> In early life periods, biology and the primary demands of reality furnish the guidelines of a necessary development. The guidelines of latency, puberty and adolescence are increasingly defined by demands of culture and sexual maturation. The adult, though, should be more or less free, even though limited by the general biological framework. In the ideal case internal processes are autonomous and are not primarily determined by immediate biological or sociocultural factors, as occurs in the preceding phases of development. (p. 139)

Such a viewpoint fails to account for the effects of aging on psychic development and minimizes the influence of such central experiences as intimacy, parenthood, work, and friendships, that is, the adult environment.

> Thus the essence of our point is that exchanges between organism and environment occur from birth to death, producing a continuous effect on psychic development. The adult is not a finished product insulated from the environment but, like the child, is in a state of dynamic tension which continually affects him. From that hypothesis a second follows. (Colarusso & Nemiroff, 1981, p. 63)

Hypothesis II. "Development in Adulthood Is an Ongoing Dynamic Process" (p. 63). This hypothesis suggests that development is continuous from birth, through childhood and adulthood, to death. The reasoning behind this hypothesis is simple enough; the body, mind, and external environment are always present and interacting. However, until recently the most prevalent thinking suggested that adults, unlike children, were not in the midst of a developmental process.

> In this instance assessment is concerned not with an ongoing process but with a finished product in which, by implication, the ultimate developmental stages should have been reached. The developmental point of view may be upheld only insofar as success or failure to reach this level or to maintain it determines the so-called maturity or immaturity of the adult personality. (A. Freud, Nagera, & W. E. Freud, 1965, p. 10)

This view of the adult, by some of the preeminent developmental thinkers of the modern era, as a finished product, outside of an ongoing developmental process, is puzzling at first glance. However, the two viewpoints may not be as diametrically opposed as they seem. The conceptual bridge between them is an increased understanding of the *difference* between the developmental process in the adult and the child, not the absence of development in the adult.

Those who propose that the developmental point of view has limited usefulness beyond adolescence seem to be saying that biological and psychological maturation and the formation of psychic structure, which are limited to childhood, are indispensable components of development. In contradistinction, adult developmentalists suggest that the aging process in the body and changes in existing psychic structures *are* the adult replacements for growth and psychic structure formation. These ideas are contained in *Hypothesis III: "Whereas Childhood Development is Focused Primarily on the Formation of Psychic Structure, Adult Development Is Concerned with the Continuing Evolution of Existing Psychic Structure and with Its Use"* (p. 65) and in *Hypothesis VI: "Development in Adulthood, as in Childhood, Is Deeply Influenced by the Body and Physical Change"* (p. 71).

Hypotheses IV and V have considerable clinical significance because they address the manner in which the therapist conceptualizes and interprets the patient's thoughts and feelings. *Hypothesis IV* states that *"The Fundamental Developmental Issues of Childhood Continue as Central Aspects of Adult Life but in Altered Form"* (p. 67). This suggests that important basic themes, such as separation–individuation processes and Oedipal phenomena, continue to affect psychic development beyond childhood and should not be understood only as significant events of the first decade of life. For example, Mahler (Winestine, 1973) described separation–individuation as a lifelong process because of the threat of loss at any time in life. The dynamic connection between the fear of loss of mother during the first 3 years and losses later in life transforms the absolute dependency on mother during childhood into a relative dependence in adulthood. We have seen (in Chapter Seven) how Blos (1967) described the transformation of separation–individuation processes in adolescence, as the *Second Individuation;* and we shall consider the matter again in Chapter Ten on young adulthood under the heading of the Third Individuation. The clinical point is that separation–individuation processes must be understood in relationship to *current* developmental tasks and conflicts, not as phenomena emanating from or exclusively related to early childhood.

Hypothesis V proposes that *"The Developmental Processes in Adulthood are Influenced by the Adult Past as Well as the Childhood Past"* (p. 69). This hypothesis implies that adult functioning and symptomatology, at any age, are an amalgam of both child and adult experience. Thus, the clinician should be as interested in the adult past as he or she is in the childhood past, determining in each instance how both sets of factors interact to produce the symptom picture and character patterns seen in the present.

Taken together, these hypotheses address the issue of reductionism in therapy and the tendency to understand all behavior in the context of the developmental phenomena of the first 5 or 6 years of life. This deeply ingrained way of thinking may be traced historically to the early focus on the Oedipal complex and then the preoedipal years. With the advent of a complimentary theory of adult development, it is now possible to recognize early childhood as the source of both personality development and pathology, but not the only, or in some instance, the most important determinant of adult pathology. A careful developmental history of childhood and adulthood will help the clinician determine the relative impact of experiences from *all* developmental phases.

Hypothesis VII addresses one of the most powerful organizers of adult experience. *"A Central, Phase-Specific Theme of Adult Development Is the Normative Crisis Precipitated by the Recognition and Acceptance of the Finiteness of Time and the Inevitability of Personal Death"* (p. 75). There is little in the anabolic thrust of childhood which directs attention to thoughts of personal death. In addition, humans show an unmistakable tendency to avoid thinking about death, to eliminate it from life (Freud, 1915). The first realization of a lengthening past occurs at the end of adolescence (Colarusso, 1988; Seton, 1974), but is quickly denied by the idealism of youth; an attempt, says Jacques (1965), to deny the "two fundamental features of human life—the inevitableness of eventual death, and the existence of hate and destructive impulses inside each person" (p. 505).

By middle adulthood these defensive maneuvers begin to break down as physical signs of aging become more obvious, parents die, and children become adults. Furthermore, there is a growing recognition that all of life's goals and ambitions will not be realized because time is running out.

The term *normative crisis* implies the inevitability, centrality, and potentially growth-promoting aspect of facing ideas of time limitation and personal death. Although difficult to do and painful, the midlife integration of the realization that one will die can be a positive developmental stimulus, prompting a reappraisal of interests, relationships, and priorities and a heightened focus on what is deemed to be truly important and valuable—while there is still time to change.

Awareness of the intrapsychic importance of time limitation and personal death is extremely important for the clinician working with individuals in middle and late adulthood because it provides an understanding of a constellation of thoughts and feelings which underlie symptoms and pathological actions—and helps the therapist come to terms with his or her own issues on this subject. In many therapeutic interactions, the subjects of time limitation and personal death are never discussed because of the unconscious collusion between patient and therapist, both of whom are avoiding the issues. Pearl King (1980) suggested that this is one of the reasons that many therapists avoid working with older patients.

TWO CONTROVERSIES

The view that development does occur in adulthood is challenged by two current theoretical controversies which question the importance of certain determinants and challenge the idea that aging and development are compatible ideas.

The Influence of Biological versus Psychological Factors

The recent rise of biological psychiatry has led to an unsophisticated polarization and adherence to either biological or psychological variables as the primary causative agents in normal development and psychopathology. Taking Spitz's definition of development into account, it is clear that any theory which discounts either biological or psychological determinants is lacking (Nemiroff & Colarusso, 1990, p. 98).

Increasingly, scholars of both disciplines are attempting an integration. In reviewing Reiser's book, *Mind, Brain and Body* (1984), Kandel (1986) commented:

> Among the most important tasks facing psychoanalysis as an evolving intellectual discipline is to develop an effective interaction with the behavioral and biological sciences: with cognitive psychology on the one hand, and with cell and molecular neurobiology on the other. (p. 36)

Approaching the issue from the viewpoint of psychoanalysis in "Will Neurobiology Influence Psychoanalysis?" Cooper (1985) wrote:

> Neurobiological research has begun to elucidate brain mechanisms of affective state and behaviorial patterns. Discussions of anxiety and sexual identity demonstrate how these researchers lead the psychoanalysts to broader views of behaviors that were previously considered psychological in origin.... Psychoanalytic theory is challenged to account for newer findings in biology and to provide important questions for further research. (pp. 1395–1402)

The balanced viewpoint which is evident in Spitz's definition did not begin with him; it originated with Freud. In his paper, "The Dynamics of Transference" (1912) he addressed the issue directly:

> I take this opportunity of defending myself against the mistaken charge of having denied the importance of innate (constitutional) factors because I have stressed that of infantile impressions ... people prefer to be satisfied with a single causative factor. Psychoanalysis has talked a lot about the accidental factors in aetiology and little about the constitutional ones; but that is only because it was able to contribute something fresh to the former, while, to begin with, it knew no more than was commonly known about the latter. We refuse to posit any contrast in principle between the two sets of aetiological factors; on the contrary, we assume that the two sets regularly act jointly in bringing about the observed result. Endowment and chance determine a man's fate— rarely or never one of those powers alone. (p. 99)

The Effect of Aging

Now let us address the issue of the effect of aging, that is, physical regression, since it is clearly the dominant biological influence in adulthood. I suggest that the aging process is as powerful an influence on adult development as growth is on child development (Colarusso & Nemiroff, 1981). The opposing view has been expressed most recently by Phyllis and Robert Tyson (1990) in their book on *Psychoanalytic Theories of Development.*

> We agree that changes occur throughout the life cycle and that certain major life events (such as marriage and parenthood or a traumatic experience of loss) serve as stimuli for psychic reorganization. But we maintain that a maturational pull (or push) is central to the developmental process. In our view, the psychological changes that come about *in* step with maturation are distinguished by psychic structure formation, differentiation, and integration. The maturational pull is not present in adult life in the same way that it is in childhood and adolescence, and so the structural changes that do occur after adolescence are mostly related to adaptation; reorganization of existing psychic structures is involved, but not the formation of new structures. (p. 15)

Settlage, Curtis, and Lozoff (1988) expressed a similar idea. "We wish to reiterate that the loss of function due to biological decline and adaptation through regression to earlier, previously developed modes of functioning does not fit our definition of development" (p. 366).

I respond to these ideas as follows. In regard to Settlage's view, when I suggest that the aging process is as powerful an influence on adult development as growth is on child development, I am not including diminished mental functioning due to organic pathology in the brain or the body. Such organic decline, particularly in the brain, will most certainly produce diminished psychological functioning. Nor do I mean regression to earlier modes of functioning.

Agreeing with the Tysons' statement, which seems to be a reiteration of Anna Freud's idea that development is synonymous with the formation of psychic structure, I accept the idea that no new psychic structures are formed in adulthood.

But in contradistinction, what is missing in both of these criticisms is the idea that the *awareness* of the adult experience of aging and the *preoccupation* with time limitation and personal death which accompanies it are increasingly powerful conscious and unconscious intrapsychic influences which grow in intensity as the young adult passes through middle age into late adulthood. They stimulate the psyche to new levels of complexity, producing intrapsychic change of such magnitude that it deserves to be called *development*.

The fact that the formation of new psychic structures is presented as an absolute prerequisite for development to occur takes into consideration Freud's early conceptualizations of developmental stage and structural theory, but ignores a growing body of theory which has emerged since then. As previously mentioned, Freud's failure to designate stages for the adult years inhibited developmental thinking for decades. A breakthrough occurred when Erikson (1963) presented his "Eight Stages of Man," extending the concept of development throughout the life cycle. Unfortunately, his series of psychological polarities only addressed one aspect of mental functioning at each developmental stage and were not followed by a more comprehensive theory of adulthood.

Building on Erikson's pioneering efforts, a strong multidetermined effort is now underway to break out of the narrow conceptualization which limits developmental processes to childhood and to elaborate a developmental theory for the years from 20 onward—for most individuals a period of time three or four times as long, and easily as important, as childhood. Evidence of significant change in psychic structure in adulthood is now very well confirmed by numerous multidisciplinary findings. Among the most prominent are the studies of Vaillant (1977) on the increasing use of mature defenses in adulthood; the longitudinal Berkeley Guidance and Oakland Growth Studies (Block, 1971), which describe the elaboration of intelligence and character structure in adulthood; and the Levinson *et al.* (1978) work on the alternating intervals of intrapsychic stability and transition which result from basic changes in the nature of the adult development process.

After reviewing these and other studies of adulthood, the eminent psychoanalytic researcher Robert Emde (1985) concluded:

> First and foremost, we must realize that the developmental thrust is not over in adolescence—far from it. There is a continuing dynamic process, and the adult personality continues to undergo structural change. Furthermore, there appears to be phase-specific aspects of this process . . . it may be, in fact, that the psychology of adult development is as important for clinical psychoanalysis as is the psychology of early development. (p. 109)

CONCEPTUALIZING DEVELOPMENT IN ADULTHOOD

Child development is organized around the familiar developmental stages—oral, anal, Oedipal, latency, and adolescence. However, the use of stages to describe development in adulthood presents some conceptual problems. For instance, if we use Erikson's (1963) division of adulthood into 20-year blocks of time, each adult phase is as long as all five childhood phases together. Furthermore, in adulthood most developmental themes do not appear with the chronological precision or the phase-specificity that they do in childhood. The developmental milestones of infancy occur within a few weeks or months. The subphases of intrapsychic processes as described by Mahler's separation–individuation theory or Piaget's cognitive developmental sequences cover months or a few years at most. By contrast, the experience of biological fatherhood may happen at any age from 13 to 80, and the intrapsychic effects will vary markedly depending on the phase of development in which it occurs.

In attempts to encompass these differences, new theoretical models are beginning to appear. In two well-known books published in 1978, Gould and Levinson *et al.* retained Erikson's division of adulthood into eras spanning 20 years, but broke them into subphases defined by false assumptions (Gould) or alternating intervals of stability and transition (Levinson). More recently, Settlage *et al.* (1988) abandoned stage theory, replacing it with the concept of *developmental process*. Developmental interactions throughout the life cycle are conceived as resulting in formation of structure and successively higher levels of organization. Through internalization and identification, the regulatory and adaptive functions and the values of important persons become parts of one's own psychic structure. The sequence is initiated by a developmental challenge, such as the need for a new skill or revision of values. This creates developmental tension, which acts as a motivating force and produces developmental conflict, reflecting normal uncertainty about change. Resolution of the developmental conflict leads to integration and internalization of the new function. The end result is a change in the individual's sense of self and identity.

Based on extensive clinical experience and a detailed knowledge of child development and object relations theory, these ideas by Settlage *et al.* not only illustrate how structural change occurs in adulthood, but also add a needed dimension to our ability to understand normal and pathological developmental processes throughout the life cycle. But like the concept of adult developmental phases, developmental process theory is not precise enough to define those experiences which shape the evolving mind in adulthood. I believe this is accomplished most effectively at present by utilizing the concept of *adult developmental tasks* (Colarusso & Nemiroff, 1981)—the psychological response to major life experiences (such as work achievement, parenthood, grandparenthood, death of loved ones, and retirement) which produce intrapsychic change as the result of actual occurrence or psychological consideration by all persons in a particular age group. When integrated with the concept of adult developmental tasks, developmental phase and developmental process theory can be usefully utilized to enrich understanding of the effect of past and present experiences on the evolving mind.

CHAPTER 9

The Adult Developmental Diagnostic Process

In Chapter Two, we considered how to utilize developmental concepts in the diagnostic evaluation of children. Now let us extend the discussion of diagnostic procedures to the adult, once again focusing on the influence of developmental thinking. Many of the concepts in this chapter are elaborations of ones first presented in Chapter 11 of *Adult Development* (Colarusso & Nemiroff, 1981). In addition to the example of a completed diagnostic workup presented at the end of this chapter, other examples on adults of various ages may be found in Chapters 6, 7, 8, 9, and 10 in *The Race against Time* (Nemiroff & Colarusso, 1985).

PURPOSE AND COMPONENT PARTS

The purpose of doing an adult developmental diagnostic evaluation is to collect relevant data about the patient which will allow the clinician to formulate a clear understanding of the normal and deviant developmental influences from childhood and adulthood which underlie the patient's healthy growth and symptomatology, and to formulate a treatment plan.

The procedures differ from those utilized with the child because the adult is qualitatively different, in most instances capable of providing the information required on his or her own. However, when pathology is extremely severe, for example, a psychosis in young or middle-aged adults or marked organicity in the elderly, other family members or interested individuals are included in the diagnostic process.

The component parts of the evaluation are the same as those utilized with children.

1. A history and mental status examination, obtained directly from the patient in most instances, or from others when the patient is incapable of participation. The information is subdivided into identifying information, chief complaint(s), history of the present illness, developmental history, and family history.
2. Additional procedures such as medical evaluations and/or psychological testing.
3. Diagnostic impressions.
4. Treatment planning.
5. A summary conference(s) in which the findings are presented.

RATIONALE AND PROCEDURES

Diagnostic Interviews. After describing the steps to be followed during the evaluation, the diagnostician encourages the nonpsychotic patient to talk about his or her concerns.

By allowing the patient to initially determine the subject matter to be discussed and the manner of its presentation, the clinician enhances the patient's comfort and cooperation. Drawing upon his or her knowledge of child and adult development, the diagnostician immediately begins to assess the relationships of both infantile and adult themes to the patient's symptomatology. For instance, depressive symptomatology in a young adult may be related to a parental divorce at age 8, feelings of inferiority during adolescence, and a broken engagement in the present. Gradually, clarifying questions are asked until the clinician can describe each symptom clearly, follow its course from inception to the present, and begin to understand the etiological factors involved.

Frequently the presenting complaints may be a direct expression of adult developmental concerns. Examples: "I've dated a lot of men and I want to get married but I'm afraid. What if I make a mistake?" or "I thought I'd enjoy being retired but I'm bored. My life doesn't have a purpose anymore."

The developmental history provides the information necessary to understand the meaning of the presenting symptoms and appreciate their effect on this unique individual. Without a detailed knowledge of the patient's life experiences, the diagnostician is reduced to making educated guesses in an impersonal context, which is an unsatisfying experience for both patient and therapist. Relying on his or her knowledge of child and adult development, the clinician traces the individual's life experience from conception to the present, relating the findings to the information obtained in the history of the present illness. The suggested outline of the child developmental history presented in Chapter Two is extended further to include the adult developmental phases described later in this chapter.

The family history provides vital data about both organic and environmental factors. In some instances, such as with manic-depressive disease, the recognition of the importance of genetic and biological factors is the key to making the correct diagnosis; while in others, environmental patterns may be most important, such as the multigenerational repetition found in child abuse.

The influence of such important figures as parents, siblings, and grandparents does not end with adolescence, because family relationships (as well as others from childhood) continue to have a major influence on psychic development throughout the adult years as well. Consequently, the course of these interactions may be traced throughout life, focusing on such critical issues as the interactions between newly married children and their middle-aged parents. Even after death, parents remain important intrapsychic objects and may be the subject of meaningful therapeutic dialogue when the clinician recognizes their importance to the older patient and inquires about them.

Additional Procedures.   Because of the preoccupation with the aging body and the increased incidence of illness and disease in middle and late adulthood, special attention should be paid to the elaboration of attitudes about the body and the determination of the presence or absence of organic disease. In many instances, patients will avoid this area and resist attempts by the diagnostician to gather information or make referrals for testing and evaluation. Unless the therapist has come to terms with the aging process in his or her own body, he or she may unconsciously collude with the patient in the avoidance. Involvement in the management of organic conditions is a critical aspect of the psychotherapeutic work with some patients. Pertinent examples may be found in the case histories presented by Gary Levinson and Gene Cohen in *The Race against Time* (Nemiroff & Colarusso, 1985).

Diagnostic and Treatment Formulations and Summary Conferences. Formulation of a diagnosis and treatment plan is conducted in the same manner as it was with a child (see Chapter Two). The clinician takes and organizes all the relevant data along descriptive, dynamic, and developmental lines. As with children, treatment recommendations take into account intrapsychic and environmental realities. If the evaluation process has gone well, the patient listens to the diagnostician's words with an awareness of the clinician's sensitivity, interest, and detailed knowledge of the patient's life experience, thus increasing the chances of acceptance of the recommendations.

RECORDING THE DATA

The following outline provides an organized approach to recording the data collected and a rationale for doing so. Of course, as described in Chapter Two, this format should be modified to suit the particular form of presentation being made—a summary conference with the patient, oral presentation to colleagues, or a formal scientific paper. Particular attention will be paid to the section on collecting the developmental history. Clinicians who are taking adult developmental histories for the first time may find the outline of questions to be asked particularly useful while they are increasing their knowledge of normal and pathological processes and developing an interviewing style of their own.

Identifying Information

1. Patient's name, age, occupation, and description.
2. Spouse or partner's name, age, occupation, and description.
3. Children's names, ages, occupations, relationship to (natural, adopted, or step) and involvement with parents.
4. Length and viability of marriage(s) or relationships.

Referral Source

In addition to serving as a reminder to thank the referring person or agency, knowledge of the manner in which the patient came to treatment—referred by self, spouse, or family physician—may provide valuable information about the patient's motivation and problems.

Chief Complaints

1. In the patient's words.
2. When relevant, in the words of other family members.
3. In the words of the referral source if other than the patient or family.

History of the Present Illness

Each symptom should be presented descriptively and chronologically. When did it begin? How has it changed over time? What makes it better or worse? Describing the symptoms in relationship to current developmental tasks and themes may be particularly useful.

Mental Status Examination

A formal mental status examination should be recorded here or at some other place in the written or oral presentation.

Developmental History

> In taking a developmental history we are learning about the past in order to relate it to the person's present and future. An in-depth, dynamic understanding of symptoms and behavior is impossible without a knowledge of those factors in the life experience of this particular individual that cause him to think and act the way he does. (Colarusso & Nemiroff, 1981, p. 195)

The following developmental history outline for the adult years is a continuation of the one for childhood and adolescence described in Chapter Two.

Young Adulthood: Ages 20–40. How does the patient feel about the aging process in his or her body? Is the body being cared for or neglected?

What is the current relationship with parents? Has an adult-to-adult relationship of mutuality and respect evolved and been expanded to include spouse and grandchildren?

Has gradually increasing sexual experience led to a sense of comfort with the body as a sexual instrument and the emergence of the capacity for intimacy?

Has childhood been recognized as a part of the past? Has a beginning acknowledgment of time limitation and personal death begun to appear? How is the female patient in her thirties reacting to the impending loss of the capacity to procreate?

Has narcissism been tempered enough to permit the evolution of a mutually gratifying relationship with a spouse and a nurturing one with children?

Has a career choice been made? Is work meaningful and enjoyable? Have mentors been utilized to facilitate this process?

Have old friendships been maintained but subordinated to the needs of spouse and children? Have new friendships, particularly with other couples, been formed?

Has play continued to be a source of pleasure, realistically tempered by the demands of work, family, and the slowly aging body?

Is money being utilized realistically to realize young adult goals, such as beginning a household, providing contemporary pleasures, and planning for the future?

What is the level of participation in religious and community activities?

Middle Adulthood: Ages 40–60. How has the aging process in the body been accepted? Is the mourning process for the body of youth identifiable? Is the body being cared for and attended to in sickness and health?

Is the idea of time limitation and personal death being accepted as an intrapsychic reality? Is this recognition acting as a positive developmental stimulant or as a source of pathology?

Is the nature of the relationship with elderly parents caring or neglectful? What was the reaction to the death of a parent?

Has intimacy and an active sexual life been maintained in the face of diminished sexual drive, menopause, and the environmental pressures of midlife?

Has an adult-to-adult relationship been forged with grown children and their spouses?

Have grandchildren been recognized and enjoyed?

Has generativity become a central aspect of relationships with all younger individuals?

Have new friendships been formed and old ones intensified, as partial replacements for grown children?

Is work a continuing source of satisfaction? Is the role of mentor being utilized to facilitate the advancement of younger colleagues? Is retirement being considered and planned for?

Is money being utilized for current pleasure, retirement planning, and the enhancement of children and society?

Late Adulthood: Ages 60 and beyond. Is body integrity being maintained through exercise and diet? Is physical infirmity and permanent impairment being accepted without diminishing the continuation of physical activity which is still possible?

Has the idea of personal death been accepted with a shift of focus to how one will die, not if one will die?

What is the reaction to the death of spouse, friends, and relatives? Are new relationships being formed to take their places?

Is there continued interest in the present and future while the life review (Butler & Lewis, 1977, Chapter 12) is being conducted?

Has the reversal of roles with children and grandchildren been accepted?

Has sexual activity been maintained when a partner is available or sexual interest and masturbation continued when one is not?

Is time invested in meaningful relationships, work, and play?

Is available money being used to care for the self and to enhance the lives of loved ones and society?

Is the life review leading to a sense of integrity and authenticity rather than despair?

Each of the areas in the developmental history may also be explored by utilizing the concept of *adult developmental lines* (Colarusso & Nemiroff, 1981). This more detailed approach to each of the areas in the developmental history will be elaborated on in the chapters on adulthood. The reader may also refer to Chapter 11 in *Adult Development* (Colarusso & Nemiroff, 1981).

Family History

This section should describe those organic and environmental factors which help explain the patient's symptoms and provide data on current support systems and sources of ongoing conflict.

Additional Procedures

An awareness of the integrity of the body and particularly the central nervous system is important in the understanding of a patient of any age, but particularly so with older patients. Relevant medical and psychological testing and other data should be presented here along with information on medications and the involvement of physicians and other physical care managers.

Diagnostic Impressions and Treatment Planning

After gathering this body of detailed information about the patient, the clinician is in a position to formulate his or her thinking along several lines, any or all of which may be emphasized depending upon the purpose of the presentation.

Using the latest edition of the *Diagnostic and Statistical Manual of Mental Disorders* of the American Psychiatric Association (1987), the clinician may arrive at a *descriptive formulation*. Such a diagnosis is useful in communicating information to other clinicians and in planning treatment regimens for well-defined conditions which are treated chemotherapeutically. However, it provides no details about the life experiences or intrapsychic state of the individual. This information can be integrated by adding a dynamic and a developmental formulation to the descriptive diagnosis.

The *dynamic formulation* provides an in-depth description of the patient's intrapsychic world by describing his or her innermost thoughts and feelings. Utilizing Freud's topographical (conscious and unconscious) and structural (id, ego, and superego) models allows the diagnostician to describe the impulses and defenses which underlie the patient's conflicts and symptoms.

The *developmental formulation* relates the patient's symptoms to past and present experiences which played a part in their formation and to those developmental processes which were, and are being, impacted.

Through the use of these three formulations, the uniqueness of each patient is appreciated and he or she comes alive to both presentor and audience. Treatment planning is also facilitated since the patient has been approached as a biopsychosocial being, thus recognizing the need to consider those psychological pharmacological, and medical procedures which will address the patient's needs.

Summary Presentation

Armed with these formulations the clinician is prepared to present his or her understanding of the patient's problems to the individual, family members, physicians, and other mental health professionals, and to treat the patient with a sense of confidence and competence which results from the completion of a thorough diagnostic evaluation.

CASE EXAMPLE

In addition to illustrating many of the concepts just presented, the following case example will serve as an introduction to diagnostic and therapeutic work with the elderly, a subject which will be discussed in more detail in Chapter Twelve, Late Adulthood. The case report also appears as part of a chapter on the "Impact of Adult Developmental Issues on Treatment of Older Patients" by Robert Nemiroff and myself in a recent book *New Techniques in the Psychotherapy of Older Patients*, edited by Wayne Myers (1991, pp. 245–265).

The information for the case study was gathered in two 45-minute sessions with Mr. A.'s children and three individual sessions with the patient.

History

Identifying Information. The patient was an 83-year-old male whose wife of 63 years had died 6 months before. A retired accountant, Mr. A. lived alone in the house he and his wife had purchased 35 years before.

He had two married children, aged 60 and 58, who lived nearby. They made the initial contact.

Chief Complaint. "Dad is forgetful. He isn't eating properly, and he's never gotten over Mom's death. We think he needs help but he doesn't want to come to see you."

History of the Present Illness. The patient's symptoms of depression and withdrawal began about 2 years ago, at the time that his wife's health began to decline seriously. His depression (clearly reactive in nature) intensified as she became sicker and reached a peak after her death. "I really miss Rose. Taking care of her was hard. I hated seeing her suffer. Now that she's gone I don't know what to do with myself." A weight loss of 40 pounds was more recent, only becoming obvious during the 6 months since his wife's death. "I don't have much of an appetite, but when I do there isn't much worth eating in the house. Rose did all the cooking." In contrast to his children's opinion, Mr. A. did not feel he was forgetful. "I'm not forgetful. I'm just not interested in much these days. I spend a lot of time with my thoughts of Rose and what our life used to be like." Various attempts by Mr. A.'s children to get him to eat and "cheer up" were unsuccessful. They were afraid to leave him alone any longer, but he refused all attempts to get him to move into one of their homes or to a nursing home.

Developmental History. Each developmental phase, from birth onward, was explored with Mr. A. and his children. Childhood phases, considered in detail in Chapter Two, will be summarized; relevant adult developmental history will be considered more fully.

Childhood. Mr. A. was an only child, born into an intact family. There was no evidence of significant physical problems at any point in childhood. His mother was involved in his care full time in infancy and early childhood. The patient was not a bed wetter, but did recall being told that he sucked his thumb until age 8. He was a good student in elementary school and had many friends. In high school he "played football, dated girls, and studied, in that order." The one traumatic event in childhood, which he recalled vividly, was the sudden death of his mother when he was 8 years old. "It took me a long time to get over that." His father remarried when the patient was 10. He had a "good" relationship with his stepmother, who died 3 years ago.

Young Adulthood (20–40). Mr. A. married his college sweetheart at age 20. After graduation, he went to work for a large accounting firm, continuing there for 15 years. At age 35 he started his own business and developed a mild depression (untreated) when the business failed. His marriage, "a very good one," was at the center of his emotional life during young and middle adulthood. Mr. A. enjoyed his children, who were born when he was in his 20s, but he and they described him as an uninvolved father. Mr. A.'s major hobby was golf. He was good at it and it consumed much of his free time, to the dismay of his wife and children. His children described him as "a physical fitness nut before there were any."

Middle Adulthood (40–60). Both children recalled Mr. A.'s depression at age 55 when their mother developed cancer. He refused treatment and the depression lifted spontaneously when his wife recovered. His children described their father's attachment to his wife as "total." The couple was very close, almost to the exclusion of their children, now grown up, and friends. Mr. A.'s involvement with his grandchildren was cordial and occasional, not unlike his relationship with his offspring when they were young. After his business failed, Mr. A. took a job with an accounting firm, remaining there in a middle-management position until he retired at age 65. He described his work as "a job. I made my try for the big bucks and I failed, so I settled for less." His physical health remained excellent throughout his adult years. In fact, he had never been hospitalized in his 83 years.

Late Adulthood (60–Present). Mr. A. liked retirement and spent his time at home with his wife or playing golf. His interest in friends and family did not increase along with his free time. "I was content to stay at home with Rose," he said, "I never needed much more than that." This pattern continued until his wife's final illness and death.

Family History. As previously described, Mr. A. was an only child, raised by loving, middle-class parents. His mother's death when he was age 8 changed his attitude toward life although it apparently did not produce symptoms. After he left home for college, he maintained a distant but cordial relationship with his father, stepmother, and half-brother until his father died when Mr. A. was 45. After that, he had even less involvement with his stepmother and half-brother.

Additional Procedures

Mr. A. refused both medical evaluation and psychological testing. He was concerned about his weight loss, but preferred to eat more rather than be evaluated. He did not plan to begin psychotherapy and saw no reason for psychological testing.

Diagnostic Impression

Descriptive. DSM III-R Dysthymia 300.40.

Dynamic. Mr. A. was deeply traumatized by the sudden death of his mother when he was 8. He used the defense mechanisms of repression and isolation to avoid the mourning process and withdrew from close emotional involvement with others until he met his wife. Her death was much more than a recapitulation of the childhood trauma; it disrupted his most significant object relationship, which had sustained him for 63 years. Deprived of his basic source of security and companionship, he became depressed and regressed.

Developmental Diagnosis. Mr. A. got off to an excellent start in life physically and psychologically. Loved and nurtured in infancy and childhood, he developed a solid sense of self and an intact personality. His mother's death during the latency years led to an arrest along the developmental line of separation from infantile objects. From then on, Mr. A. maintained a defensive distance from all significant objects in his life—with the exception of his wife—so as not to be hurt again. His development proceeded smoothly along most developmental lines in adolescence, and he was able to get an education, work, marry, and raise a family—but always from a protective distance. This partly adaptive, partly neurotic equilibrium continued until the death of his wife of 63 years.

Treatment Plan

Individual psychotherapy should be undertaken for Mr. A.

Try to keep Mr. A. in his home as long as he is physically able by providing him with a full-time housekeeper to cook and clean. Encourage his involvement with friends and senior organizations (which he and his wife had attended prior to her illness). Have members of the extended family be in touch on a daily basis, involving him in activities as much as possible despite his reluctance. Recognize that his need to mourn for his wife will extend for many more months because in late adulthood, particularly if the spousal relationship had existed for many years, mourning takes longer and is not the same process, qualitatively, as it is in younger people.

If the above fails, consider having Mr. A. live with either of his children, despite his reluctance.

As a last resort, Mr. A. should be considered for a nursing home.

Summary Conferences

The above recommendations were presented separately to Mr. A. and his family. The recommendations for psychotherapy and a full-time housekeeper were eventually accepted by Mr. A. Three months later, he remains in his home, has gained five pounds, and is beginning to trust the therapist enough to discuss some of his feelings about the loss of his wife. The short-term prognosis is fair to good.

CHAPTER 10

Young Adulthood (Ages 20–40)

THE SHIFT FROM BIOLOGICAL PROGRESSION
TO RETROGRESSION

Although perhaps not exclusive to it, certain experiential and biological phenomena characterize young adulthood. For example, it is the time when most individuals in Western culture leave home, begin careers, marry, and become parents. However, the shift from physical progression to retrogression, from growth to aging, is one biological phenomenon unique to this phase.

This strikingly obvious and developmentally significant event has scarcely been addressed in the literature. Sigmund Freud (1905) firmly linked maturation to development in childhood, delineating the libidinal progression from zone to zone. The conceptualization of oral, anal, Oedipal, latency, and adolescent stages was an elaboration upon this biologically determined sequence. Freud did not apply this formulation to adulthood and consequently did not explore the question of the effect of biological retrogression on adult developmental processes, an omission that impeded for several decades the emergence of theoretical interest in the relationship between aging and psychological development.

It is important to recognize that there is no interval between the end of maturational progression and the beginning of physical retrogression. The two forces overlap during young adulthood, but the aging process gradually replaces the growth process as the dominant biological influence. Evidence of this ranges from a slowing of the reflexes, loss of skin tone, and the early signs of balding (in some individuals during their 20s) to the far more dramatic loss of the procreative function in women as they approach and traverse age 40.

THE TRANSITION FROM ADOLESCENCE
TO YOUNG ADULTHOOD

The transition from adolescence to young adulthood is based on an increased capacity for real and intrapsychic separation from the family of origin and the engagement of phase-specific tasks. Blos (1979) described this process as "the shedding of family dependencies, the loosening of infantile object ties in order to become a member of society at large, or simply, of the adult world" (p. 142). Kohut (Wolf, 1980) wrote of the "transformation from preadolescent idealized parental images to the post-adolescent idealized ethics and values" (p. 48). Settlage (Panel, 1973a,b) noted the gradual shift from the family of origin to the family of procreation.

Normally this transition is tolerated and endured as a necessary time to build adult structures, both internal and external. The length of time it takes to make the intrapsychic transition from dependent child to independent adult (alone in the world, enjoying it, and not yet ready for permanent attachments to spouse and child) varies from person to person, but it must occur eventually if development is to proceed.

In his studies of individuals from the Berkeley Guidance Study and the Oakland Growth Study (long-term studies on normal development begun in 1929 and 1932, respectively), Block (1971) discovered that psychological adjustment in adulthood was not easily predicted from adjustment during adolescence. This important observation supports the idea that a current, phase-specific conflict can lead to the reworking of past conflicts with better resolutions or to the onset of pathology, which may become evident for the first time.

The same idea is incorporated by Levinson et al. (1978) in their characterization of transitions, intervals of approximately 5 years of change and turmoil, which occur between periods of relative stability. The transition from late adolescence to young adulthood occurs between the ages of 17 and 22. During these years, the individual resolves the issue of childhood dependency sufficiently to establish self-reliance. In addition, the goal is "to explore, to expand one's horizons and put off making firmer commitments until the options are clear; and to create an initial life structure, to have roots, stability, and continuity" (Levinson et al., 1978, p. 80).

Another important intrapsychic aspect of the transition is a redefinition of the childhood and adolescent past. As I have expressed it elsewhere:

> For the first time, an entire phase of life must be consigned to the past. This process, which is gradual and painful, brings closure to an epoch of life and forces a further redefinition of aspects of psychic structure, particularly the

superego and ego ideal and the self. The late adolescent can no longer think of himself as a child and so must continue the comprehensive intrapsychic reorganization that will lead to his definition as a young adult. (Colarusso, 1988, p. 191)

THE DEVELOPMENTAL TASKS OF YOUNG ADULTHOOD

Developing a Young Adult Sense of Self and Other: The Third Individuation

According to Offer and Offer (1975), "the establishment of a self separate from the parents is one of the major tasks of young adulthood" (p. 167). For most young adults, the gradual emotional detachment from parents is followed by a new inner definition of themselves as comfortably alone and competent, able to care for themselves in the real and intrapsychic worlds. This shift away from the parents continues long after marriage and parenthood produce new relationships which replace the parents as the most important individuals in the young adult's life and transform his or her inner world.

Psychological separation from the parents is followed by a second step—the synthesis of mental representations from the childhood past and the young adult present. For example, as their own children move from phase to phase, young parents reengage memories of their own childhoods, fusing their experiences as children with those of their children, and their experiences as parents with memories of their own progenitors from a generation ago. Such a conceptualization moves us beyond understanding adolescent separation as simply a "disengagement" from parents.

As described in earlier chapters, the separation–individuation process (Mahler *et al.*, 1975) is responsible in infancy for the establishment of a stable sense of self and the capacity to relate to others. Building on Mahler's work, Blos (1979) described the process of psychological separation from the parents in adolescence as a *second individuation*. I have addressed the separation–individuation process in young adulthood in some detail as the "third individuation," (Colarusso, 1990) defining it as

that continuous process of elaboration of the self and differentiation from objects which occurs in the developmental phases of young (20 to 40) and middle (40 to 60) adulthood. Although it is influenced by all important adult object ties, at its core are object ties to children, spouse, and parents, i.e., the family, the same psychological constellation that shaped the first and second individuations. (p. 181)

Adult developmental theory postulates a growing complexity in relationships as the individual moves from infancy through childhood and adolescence to adulthood. This may be depicted as an inverted pyramid. From the diagram (Figure 1) it may be seen that the first individuation is a rather exclusive affair between infant and mother (and to a lesser degree, infant and father). The base expands during the second individuation to include important nonfamilial relationships, such as friends, girlfriends and boyfriends, and mentors. They become the recipients of some libidinal and aggressive drives formerly directed toward the parents and thus facilitate the process of psychological separation from them.

The transition from the second to the third individuation is a young adult experience, stimulated by the growing capacity for intrapsychic separation from the parents and engagement of the phase-specific developmental tasks of young adulthood. Sooner or later, this psychic state drives most young adults to fill the real and intrapsychic voids left by separation from the parents of childhood by establishing a family of procreation. Various aspects of the third individuation will be described in the sections that follow dealing with the developmental tasks of intimacy, marriage, parenthood, and separating from parents.

Developing the Capacity for Intimacy: Becoming a Spouse

Erikson (1963) defined the major developmental dichotomy of his Stage VI, *young adulthood,* as *intimacy versus stagnation.* In adulthood,

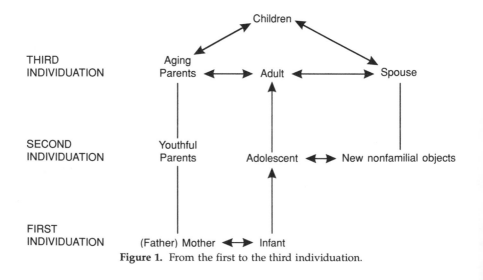

Figure 1. From the first to the third individuation.

intimacy requires one to "experience someone else's needs and concerns as equally important as one's own" (p. 31). The capacity for intimacy has its roots in the quality of early parent–child relationships, the successful resolution of the Oedipal complex, and adolescent sexual experimentation. But it does not become a *sustainable* capacity until young adulthood. As defined by Nemiroff and myself (Colarusso & Nemiroff, 1981), adult intimacy presupposes a significant relationship with a partner which is elaborated over time and usually is associated with deep emotional commitment and shared parenthood.

Offer and Offer (1975) observed in their study that the capacity for intimacy in the sense used by Erikson was apparent in the highest functioning individuals by the fourth post-high school year. It seems clear from their work and that of A. Freud (1958) and Blos (1979) that the capacity for intimacy in the adult sense is made possible by the physical, sexual, and psychological changes of adolescence.

The developmental shift from sexual experimentation to the desire for intimacy is experienced internally as an intense loneliness, resulting from the lack of close relationships with others, such as existed in childhood with the parents. Brief sexual encounters in short-lived relationships no longer serve as significant boosts to self-esteem. The young adult self has essentially mastered the task of capable sexual performance and mere repetition will no longer provide emotional satisfaction. Increasingly, the desire is for emotional connectedness in a sexual context. According to Erikson, the young adult who fails to actualize a lasting intimate relationship runs the risk of living in isolation and self-absorption in midlife.

The achievement of adult sexual intimacy produces significant intrapsychic change. Through the repeated fusion of sex and love, the self is increasingly identified with the partner. The superego may become more flexible and tolerant as sexual thoughts, feelings, and practices are repeated in relation to the esteemed partner. Feminine or masculine aspects of the self are projected onto and accepted and loved in the partner. The ego ideal is altered by the inclusion of the partner's aspirations for the couple's future, particularly in regard to the major aspects of young adult life, such as where to live, the desire for children, and career ambitions.

Another result of the development of the capacity for intimacy is acceptance of the equal status and complementary nature of the male and female genitals. Repeated experiences with foreplay, intercourse, conception, pregnancy, childbirth, and psychological parenthood—all within the framework of intimacy—provide the optimal environment in which to abandon infantile notions and replace them with the recognition that female and male genitalia are equal and interdependent for adult sexual pleasure, intimacy, and reproduction. There is a distinct parallel between the role of intimacy in childhood and in adulthood. In both, whether it is between mother and child or woman and man, intimacy is the fertile soil from which healthy development springs.

For most individuals in Western culture, intimacy leads to marriage in young childhood. Based on his analysis of longitudinal data from the Grant Study at Harvard, George Vaillant (1977) noted that there was "probably no single longitudinal variable that predicted mental health as clearly as a man's capacity to remain happily married over time" (p. 320). Referring to the views of major adult developmental theorists on marriage, Emde (1985) commented:

> There is a recognition that in a marriage each partner has to work on a restructuring; where there is commitment, marriages are stable; where there is no such a commitment to continuing in spite of restructuring, they are not stable, irrespective of troubles or turmoil. (p. 111)

Becoming a Biological and Psychological Parent

Although biological parenthood is not universal or limited to young adulthood, it is experienced by most individuals for the first time during this phase of development. To place parenthood in a developmental context, using information presented in earlier chapters, consider the developmental line of sexual identity during childhood:

1. *Oral phase*—The basic sense of maleness or femaleness—core gender identity (Stoller, 1968) is firmly established by 18 months of age.
2. *Anal phase*—By age 3, children recognize and incorporate the idea that there are two sexes (Galenson & Roiphe, 1976).
3. *Oedipal phase* —Sexuality is experienced within relationships.
4. *Latency phase*—Subjective family, community, and cultural attitudes about masculinity and femininity are integrated.
5. *Adolescence*—The maturational changes of puberty are followed by the use of the adult body as a sexual instrument, first with the self, then with others.
6. *Young adulthood*—The developmental experience of intimacy and parenthood are added.

Ritvo (1976) stated, that "in the adolescent girl the wish for a child is still strongly tinged with oedipal and preoedipal origins" (p. 135). In young adulthood, the developmental task, for both sexes, is to separate the wish for a child from its origins in the infantile relationship with the parents and to increasingly attach it to the spouse and the need to actualize the procreative purpose of the genitals, thus confirming the integrity of the body as a mature sexual instrument and realizing the expectations of the ego ideal that one will become a parent. This is not a simple or conflict-free process. Indeed, it most often creates tension within the developing young adult dyadic intimacy of marriage, as described by Kestenberg (1976):

> Entering her first adult developmental phase (Erikson, 1959) the young woman seeks intimacy with a new permanent object and is not ready for a new triangular relationship. Once the partners have become accustomed to the fact that they cannot be mother and father to each other, there is partial disillusionment and a renewal of the search for ideal closeness. Too much closeness breeds aggression, yet separation is not the solution. Planning a child, the young woman renews her position as a potential mother. By consenting to have a child, the husband reclaims the role of a masculine protector and can also sublimate his own wish to be a mother. For him, the seed that perpetuates his father and himself is no longer wasted. For the prospective mother, her inner genitals receive a confirmation and an enlargement of scope, comparable to that of the pregnant mother of her child. The conception-coitus revives oedipal feelings in both parents and allows for a reworking of the adult superego vis à vis the previously forbidden actions that led to pregnancy. (p. 227)

Hertzog (1982) related the ability to weather this powerful real and intrapsychic transition to the depth of the young couples' attachment to each other.

In his case report of a 23-year-old man, Gurwitt (1982) described the effects of the patient's wife's pregnancy:

> I propose that the period of impregnation and pregnancy constitutes an important developmental challenge for the prospective father, which like other developmental crises, brings about internal upheaval and change...these psychological events occur in the context of the special tasks of young adulthood. (p. 244)

For this patient, his wife's pregnancy initiated "a major reworking of the past and current relationships with his mother, father, siblings, and wife, as well as a shift and resynthesis of his sense of self" (p. 295). This was particularly true of Oedipal themes with the father:

> For this son to become a father like his father, yet not just like him; to become a procreator with a woman who now, more than ever before, was linked to his mother, was heavy work indeed. (p. 295)

Biological parenthood begins the process of psychological parenthood, that mental state in which healthy young adults become increasingly attached to and involved with their offspring. For both parents-to-be, pregnancy adds a new dimension to sexual identity by confirming that the sexual apparatus is capable of performing the primary function for which it was intended. After birth, each interaction with the infant enhances the new sense of sexual completeness and stimulates the desire to engage the baby who is so strongly identified with the self. When a young couple become parents for the first time, a *family* is created; its structure is identical to the family of origin except for the reversal of roles. The former child, now the parent, ministers to his own creation. As the child grows, the new parents undergo profound intrapsychic change, resulting from a simultaneous reexamination of their own experiences as children and the growing sense of themselves as adults (Colarusso, 1990).

Parenthood complicates the relationship between the new parents. Through their physical and emotional union, the couple has created a fragile, dependent being who needs them in the interlocking roles of father and mother. This recognition expands their internal representations of one another to include thoughts and feelings emanating from the role of parent. The superego and ego ideal are modified to include the concept of parenthood, and as they work together over the years, their basic senses of self become those of parents relating to one another and to their children.

Becoming a parent also stimulates further individuation from their own parents. Assuming the role that was formerly the exclusive prerogative of the progenitors leads to an inner sense of parity. Furthermore, constant conscious and unconscious comparisons between child-rearing practices heighten the internal sense of difference while they reinforce connectedness and continuity between the generations.

Finally, the ability to be instrumental in the midlife development of one's own parents by providing them with the experience of grandparenthood is striking evidence of the shift in the power balance between former child and parent and foreshadows the not-too-distant future when the elderly parent may become dependent upon his or her offspring for physical and psychological well-being.

Separating Psychologically from Parents while Facilitating Their Midlife Development

Real and intrapsychic relationships to parents undergo dramatic change during young adulthood. This process may be divided into three related phases which build upon one another.

Phase I. There is a continuing psychological separation from parents. Not all aspects of the first (Mahler) and second (Blos) individuations are resolved by the end of adolescence; both, but particularly the more recent second individuation, continue to be engaged during young adulthood. The ability to function relatively independently of intrapsychic representations of the parents of infancy and early childhood—meaning without using them as a major source of comfort, security, and direction—comes to fruition during the young adult years.

Building on the developmental achievements of adolescence, this process is greatly facilitated by the young adult creating a family of procreation. As the spouse is internalized as a source of identification and gratifier of basic needs and new objects assume roles of intrapsychic importance, the power of earlier parental introjects is gradually diminished. Modification and transformation of these childhood representations are further accomplished by their fusion with current representations of the spouse and the self in conjunction with the functions of both as spouse and parent. Every young adult brings from childhood a detailed program, largely unconscious, but firmly institutionalized in the superego/ego ideal, of how a husband or wife and parent should act. These idealized parent expectations must be modified by current reality if they are to be adaptive.

Phase II. Once the young adult has assumed and internalized the adult roles of spouse–parent–provider, the stage is set for the establishment of an inner sense of equality and mutuality with his or her parents. This occurs as the internal representations of the self-spouse gradually become qualitatively the same as those of the parents when they were young adults. As the young adult marries, has sexual relations, becomes a parent, works, buys a home, and develops adult friendships, and so forth, and as these adult experiences become the substance of everyday life, they transform the intrapsychic relationship with the representation of the parents of childhood from one of dependency and need to one of mutuality and equality.

These transformations change the real relationship with the parents and provide a powerful rationale for the young adult to remain invested in them. *Only parents and children place one in the center of a genetic continuity that spans three generations.* As we move toward middle age and a growing preoccupation with time limitation and personal death, the intrapsychic importance of this "genetic immortality" grows.

Phase III. The attainment of equality and mutuality with parents may continue throughout the remainder of young and middle adulthood, or it may be short-lived, depending on the mental and physical well-being of the parents. At some point, the adult "child" will be confronted with the psychological and possibly physical task of caring for vulnerable, dependent parents who no longer can care for themselves. When this occurs, the internal representations of the dependent, vulnerable childhood self and the aging parent are brought together in the superego/ego ideal and compared. In the normal adult, the superego demands that the "child" reenter the parent–child dyad, now reversed, and assume the role of caretaker.

Simultaneously, throughout the young adult and middle years, living parents and grandparents provide examples of how the developmental tasks of these phases may be engaged. As the young adult parent and his children internalize these examples, they lay the foundation for their own interaction in the years to come when their roles will be reversed.

This theoretical conceptualization of the interaction between grown children and their parents is supported by findings in the Berkeley Guidance Study and the Oakland Growth Study. In analyzing the massive amounts of data accumulated in those studies, Block (1971) observed that the adult personalities of children closely resembled those of one or both parents. This resemblance may be attributed not only to the earlier adult–child interaction but also to their continuing relationships as adult–adult.

Block described the influence of both parents, not just the parent of the same sex. The identification with the parent of the opposite sex actually increases in young adulthood because heterosexual identity is strengthened after marriage, particularly if it leads to psychological parenthood. The young adult is then free to identify with and incorporate valued aspects of the character of the opposite-sex parent, particularly in regard to the parent's engagement of the developmental tasks of middle and late adulthood.

FRIENDSHIPS

In late adolescence and young adulthood, before the establishment of a committed relationship and parenthood, friendships are often the primary source of emotional sustenance. In the years between the family of origin and the family of procreation, the young adult finds himself or herself in a state of relative object loss, with little opportunity for the gratification of impulses within a committed relationship. I have called this state the *loneliness of young adulthood* (Colarusso, 1990). Roommates, apartment mates, sorority sisters, and fraternity brothers, as indicated by the names used to describe them, are substitutes for family, temporary stand-ins until more permanent replacements are found and created.

The emotional needs for companionship, acceptance, and confidentiality are largely met by friendships. Sexual and aggressive issues related to dating and work are discussed with friends, particularly those in similar circumstances.

As the twenties move into the thirties, the central emotional importance of friendships is diminished, sooner or later replaced in prominence by spouse and children. Many friendships become casualties of this developmental progression since the spouse may not accept the friend, recognizing at some level that they are competitors. From the shifting and shuffling of relationships which take place at this time emerges a new form of friendship—couples friendships—which is a reflection of the new committed status but more difficult to form and maintain because four individuals must be compatible, not just two.

As children grow and begin to move into the community, the parents follow them to dance classes and little league games, thus providing the progenitors with a new focus and use of time. It also provides them with the opportunity to make friends with other parents who are at the same point developmentally and who are receptive to the formation of relationships, which helps to explain and cushion the pressures of young adult life.

WORK

The acquisition of a work identity is a central developmental task of young adulthood. When this developmental line is relatively conflict free, there is a smooth progression from high school to on-the-job training or from high school to college and sometimes beyond. The transition from learning and play to work may be gradual or abrupt, but at some point, usually in the late teens or twenties, the growth of the work identity within the superego and ego ideal leads to the recognition that work must become a central activity and the subordination of the pleasures of play and/or learning to the temporal and emotional demands of job or career. Depending upon the work itself, and attitudes toward it, work may continue to be a source of frustration, a necessary evil, or a source of pleasure and self-esteem which gradually leads to a shift in identity from child to adult and from player to worker.

One young adult female had greatly enjoyed her 5 years in college and had only reluctantly acquired a job with a large real estate firm. Somewhat of a hippie, she had limited interest in her appearance and began work in clothing borrowed from her mother and her sister. She scoffed when the boss gave her an advance to buy an upscale wardrobe, but began to enjoy the fine clothing and the respect engendered by her appearance and position. As her income began to rise, work became a source of pleasure and self-esteem and a means for acquiring the trappings of adulthood.

The young adult, regardless of the job or career, must assume the role of a protégé, working with a mentor in order to acquire information and skills and forge a work identity. The identification with the mentor is based on infantile identifications, but this adult process is not a duplication of the parent–child relationship. The relationship normally goes through three phases: first, a fusion with the mentor; then, through partial identifications, an internalization of aspects of the mentor into the self; and finally a psychological separation and further individuation.

> In the initial phase the mentor is idealized, as the internal representation of the mentor is invested with narcissism displaced from the self. The sense of fusion during the middle phase brings great pleasure but leaves the self vulnerable since the mentor's approval is necessary for a sense of well-being . . . . During the separation process considerable pain is experienced, but after a period of working through, the self emerges stronger, enhanced by the greater sense of individuation and capability. (Colarusso & Nemiroff, 1981)

Clinicians need to be aware of the importance of this developmental process and extremely sensitive to the presence—or absence—of material about work and work relationships. As will become apparent later in this chapter in the case of Jim, problems with work may be a major symptom, rooted in significant internal conflict. In other patients work may be the unrecognized source of interference with other developmental themes. For instance, a 28-year-old lawyer working 80 hours per week did not recognize that his impotence and sense of social isolation were partially due to chronic fatigue and lack of time as well as more deeply seated needs to avoid sex and intimacy.

PLAY

Young adulthood is the phase of development during which the ability to perform most of the physical games learned in childhood and adolescence reaches a peak and then declines. Some of the fantasies from childhood about athletic fame and fortune are realized but most are not, forcing a more realistic appraisal of capability and potential and a mourning for what was not achieved. Aspirations for athletic greatness are not easily relinquished, however; and some are maintained unconsciously through identification with professional star players who are now chronological contemporaries. For some, these identifications continue into middle and late adulthood—these are the true fans. For others, time, age, and the acceptance of the aging process in the middle-aged body stretch the credibility of comparisons between youthful heroes and the middle-aged self until such identifications become impossible, thus leading to a diminished interest in spectator sports and a search for new forms of play.

Although patterns of childhood play continue into the adult years, new forms of play reflecting the growing importance of spouse and children emerge. These range from physical activities with the partner to mental games, such as bridge, with friends. Encouragement of the play activities of children are a powerful source of narcissistic gratification for some, providing a second chance to realize childhood goals (often at the expense of the child) at the same time that physical decline and reality are forcing a recognition that the fantasies of childhood will not be realized.

Clinicians need to recognize that material about play is a rich source of information about childhood, the exploration of which may lead to unexpected revelation and insight. In some individuals, reactions to physical injury resulting from a failure to temper the intensity of play in keeping with the aging body may be a presenting symptom, reflecting significant intrapsychic conflicts around achievement and self-esteem.

CHANGES IN PSYCHIC STRUCTURE IN YOUNG ADULTHOOD

The literature on this subject is sparse because of the predominant idea that changes in psychic structure do not occur in adulthood; but perspectives are changing. Emde (1985), for one, stated flatly, "From a psychological standpoint, it seems clear that structural change does not stop at adolescence" (p. 60).

The Ego

In young adulthood the ego significantly increases its ability to *consistently* (1) control impulses, (2) delay gratification, (3) limit and control aggression, (4) channel energy into work and other sublimated activities, and (5) separate from infantile objects and form new loving relationships. Another way to describe some of the changes in psychic structure in young adulthood would be the use of Hartmann's (1964) term "ego interests"; namely, the focus of the young adult ego on social status, wealth, professional success, comfort, and influence.

Defenses. Some of the most influential work on changes in ego functioning in young adulthood has been done by George Vaillant (1990) as part of the Grant Study. As of 1989, the longitudinal examinations of a population of postwar Harvard undergraduates has continued for 47 years, through young adulthood and midlife. These men were twice as likely in young adulthood as in adolescence to use the mature defenses of sublimation suppression, anticipation, and humor. The change was even more dramatic in middle adulthood when mature defenses were utilized four times more frequently than in adolescence. In addition, by midlife, Vaillant's subjects were using relatively fewer immature defense mechanisms, that is, acting out, projection, hypochondriasis, and masochism.

Emde (1985) noted that major restructuring of the defenses is the usual experience in young adulthood under favorable environmental circumstances. In a similar vein, Jacques (1965) related the defensive shift toward optimism and idealism that he observed in young adults to the need to cope with growing preoccupations with the "two fundamental features of human life—the inevitableness of eventual death, and the existence of hate and destructive impulses inside each person" (p. 505).

Object Relationships. In young adulthood, for the first time, the healthy individual develops the capacity to form and maintain stable, sustaining object ties independent of the infantile objects. Vaillant (1977), Heath (1979), and Arnstein (1980) all stressed the importance of relationships in college and later life as indicators of psychological health and observed a high correlation between the ability to establish friendships then and the capacity to maintain intimate relationships in adulthood.

Intelligence. In the 1940s, Wechsler (1941) proposed that an individual's I.Q. increased into his or her 20s and then declined throughout the remainder of life. This notion has persisted despite detailed longitudinal studies, particularly those by Jarvik, Eisdofer, and Blum (1973), which convincingly demonstrate that in the presence of central nervous system intactness, intelligence increases throughout young and middle adulthood. In young adulthood, this increase is stimulated, in particular, by intense preoccupation with learning facts and acquiring new motor skills involved in becoming proficient in work or a career.

Even more fascinating are new post-Piagetian ideas about intelligence in adulthood. Like Freud, Piaget ended his construct of a developmental line with adolescence, describing attainment of the capacity for abstraction as the highest order of thinking. Now, however, the nature of thought in adulthood is being described as far more complex. Commons and Richards (1982) have extended Piaget's construct to include a stage beyond formal operations. They call it *structural analytic thought,* and with it the young adult thinker begins to grasp the connectedness between sets of relationships, in other words, the relationships between systems. A similar conclusion is reached by Basseches (1984) in his conceptualization of dialectical thinking. Although formal thinkers focus on universals, dialectical thinkers are relativists, recognizing that interactions exist among ideas and facts which create "truth" within a particular system of thought or historical period. Contradiction and paradox are pathways to new ideas and synthesis which themselves are immediately subject to critique and change.

Another theorist, Gisela Labouvie-Vief (1982a,b) suggested that some young and middle-aged adults progress beyond both formal operations and dialectical thought to the stage she calls *autonomous thought*. Whereas the formal operational thinker can analyze relationships within a finite, closed system and the dialectical thinker can recognize that some truths are relevant only within particular systems, the autonomous thinker integrates logical and irrational aspects of experience and understands that the thinker participates in the creation of truth. Further cognitive development beyond adolescence is also suggested by the work of Rybash, Hoyer, and Roodin (1986). They believe that thought becomes increasingly relative in adulthood, because of the newly emergent ability to synthesize experience and emotional and contradictory thought. Change in the nature of thought does not end in early adulthood. Chinen (1984) and others have considered the evolving nature of thought in middle and late adulthood. These ideas will be presented in Chapter Twelve on late adulthood.

Reality Testing. The ability to test and comprehend reality grows in complexity and capacity in young adulthood. This is due to: (1) greater awareness of and comfort with the inner world, that is, sexual and aggressive impulses, resulting in less tendency to distort internal and external stimuli; (2) greater experience in living, leading to increased capacity to manage everyday events autonomously and with less stress—as A. Freud (1981) put it, with "full cognizance of the importance of cause and effect" (p. 130); (3) a qualitative increase in the ability to think and reason which enhances the synthetic function of the ego; and (4) engagement of phase-specific developmental tasks, such as the growing awareness of time limitation and personal death.

For many individuals, the continued elaboration of all these ego functions, when coupled with the experience in living gained during young and middle adulthood, results in enhanced capacity for introspection and the emergence of *wisdom*, that special ability to understand and interpret human experience from the vantage point of the second half of life.

The Superego and the Ego Ideal

The *superego* and the *ego ideal* are terms used to describe those aspects of the personality that deal with the judgment of thought and behavior (superego) and ideal expectation of the self in the present and the future (ego ideal). In young adulthood, these psychic agencies must adapt to changes in the body, mind, and external environment which stimulate the need to establish independent functioning, new relationships, adult sexual life, and a work identity.

At the beginning of young adulthood, this involves a loosening of childhood restrictions and attitudes to allow for greater freedom to think and experience. For example, Katz (1968) found that college students "lessen previous constrictive and restrictive controls over their own impulses, and adopt more tolerant and permissive attitudes toward the behavior of others" (p. 5). Conversely and paradoxically, the superego/ego ideal must also deal with the realistic need to narrow choices, abandoning many of the unattained goals from childhood and adolescence without undue guilt or excessive mourning while gratifying the self for successful choices made and achievements realized.

The tension between these two paradoxical trends leads to normative conflict which gradually produces what Ritvo (1976) called a more "reality-attuned ego ideal" (p. 128), one based primarily on young adult and middle adult experience and trends rather than infantile fantasy.

Because of increased awareness of physical aging and the increased complexity of relationships in young adulthood, there is a growing preoccupation with an uncertain future. As Neugarten (1979) commented:

> It is often said that the task for the young adult is to undertake one's anticipated life script while accepting the reality that the script will be continually altered in ways that cannot be predicted and that can only be partially controlled. (p. 890)

In addition, the future is experienced very differently at the beginning and end of the young adult years. In the early 20s, it is long and open-ended. Although, as Neugarten pointed out, future sense is filled with uncertainty and unpredictability, there remains plenty of time to meet the demands of the superego/ego ideal in regard to mastering young adult developmental tasks; hence in the normative situation, when satisfactory progress is being made with regard to work, separation from parents, and establishing new object ties, there is little conflict between the ego and the superego/ego ideal. By the late 30s, a very different attitude toward the future begins to be realized through a gradual shift from time lived to time left-to-live. The past is increasingly seen as long and layered when compared to the future. Many major aspects of adult life have been engaged, successfully or otherwise. Gradually, the future becomes a time to anticipate limited opportunity at work (Bardwick, 1986), heavy responsibility at home, and aging and illness.

To summarize, the young adult superego/ego idea is dealing with how well the internalized expectations from childhood and adolescence are realized, the integration of young adult demands for instinctual gratification and control, and the preparation of expectations for future developmental stages. The result of this profound, ongoing intrapsychic reorganization is the emergence of a psychic agency that regulates self-esteem independent of the parents and that facilitates "the development of a personally acceptable code of behavior which is potentially satisfying to the individual . . . [and is] . . . constant with external reality" (Arnstein, 1980, p. 137).

FEMALE DEVELOPMENT IN YOUNG ADULTHOOD

A radical change in the psychodynamic theory of female development was crystallized in 1976 when the *Journal of the American Psychoanalytic Association* devoted an entire supplement to the topic of Female Psychology. As a foundation for our consideration of young adulthood, let us review some of the ideas from this supplement which were presented earlier. Female development was conceptualized as having its own line of development from birth onward; Freud had proposed that male and female psychic development were identical until the Oedipal phase. Furthermore, penis envy was no longer seen as the core of female development during the Oedipal phase. The normal girl was regarded as entering late adolescence with a firmly established sense of femininity and an awareness of the complementary nature of the male and female genitalia. The journal supplement was also noteworthy because it extended the consideration of female development into the adult years. Ritvo (1976), for example, discussed young adult womanhood in the following terms:

> In sexual life the woman will have established or be well on the way to genital responsiveness in a mutually satisfying relationship. She will be capable to entering into, maintaining, and deriving satisfaction from a lasting and stable relationship, capable of surviving the average expectable stresses of daily living. She will have articulated these with a reality-attuned ego ideal, which will include the image of herself as mother, as well as her own place in the community in whatever other capacity she has chosen and achieved. This is obviously an unattainable idealized prescription, but it will serve as a conceptual guide. (p. 128)

Included in that statement are some of the major developmental tasks and issues with which all young adult women must deal intrapsychically, if not in actuality.

Aspirations for a career and motherhood are particularly pressing issues for many young women. The freedom that women experience today, when there is no single socially prescribed role for them, provides opportunities for both growth and development and for considerable inner turmoil (Ticho, 1976). Clinicians are seeing increasing numbers of disillusioned young adult women—and men—who concentrated on their careers in their 20s and 30s and did not marry and have children. They are usually very accomplished in the workplace, but often lonely, depressed, and bitter. By focusing exclusively on their careers, they ignored the vital, *time-limited*, phase-specific young adult developmental tasks of marriage and parenthood. The biologically determined loss of procreative capacity in females in their 30s and early 40s is the most striking developmental difference between the sexes in young adulthood, affecting almost every other developmental line.

Clinical Vignette: A childless 38-year-old, divorced lawyer sought couples therapy for herself and her live-in boyfriend of 2 years. She wanted to marry and have children, but he was unsure of his commitment to the relationship. She had become increasingly anxious and depressed over the past several years, and was aware that the passage of time was diminishing her chances to have children.

A basic tenet of dynamic child development theory states that psychopathology results from failure to engage in and master major developmental tasks during the phase of development in which they are central issues. This is equally true in adulthood. An understanding of the basic biological and psychological forces that underlie normal young adult development may also provide individuals in this phase and their clinicians with the knowledge needed to prevent such young adult psychopathology.

The following sequence is presented as a developmental guideline which might be followed by women in young adulthood as they attempt to simultaneously engage the three major developmental tasks of career, marriage, and parenthood.

1. Pursue education and career choice in the late teens and the 20s and continue into the 30s when indicated (e.g., in residency training or other postgraduate education).
2. Marry *during* this process, ideally during the 20s, when most young adults are psychologically ready and are looking for mates.
3. Have children before the middle 30s, well within the bounds of biologically determined readiness and ability. While the child is

under the age of 3, work or train on a part-time basis to promote the healthy development of the child and enjoy the experience of motherhood.

4. Return to full-time career status when children are in school.

This scheme is presented as a guideline, which like all guidelines, must be fitted to individual circumstances. However, as at any other point in the life cycle, ignorance of the developmental processes involved, or failure to seriously consider and engage them, is likely to produce negative consequences.

CLINICAL ILLUSTRATIONS

In this section the treatment of two men will be presented in order to demonstrate the clinical usefulness of the theory just presented and to illustrate some aspects of male development in young adulthood, particularly the relationship between son and father. The first patient was a young man of 25, struggling to make the transition from adolescence. The second patient was a man of 35, who was trying to live with the consequences of his young adult actions as he approached middle age.

Jim

The evaluation of Jim when he was a child was presented in Chapter Two on the diagnostic process in childhood. As mentioned there, a detailed description of his childhood treatment was recently published in *Psychoanalytic Case Studies* (Sholevar and Glenn, 1991). Thirteen years later, Jim returned to treatment, thus allowing us to trace his development into young adulthood.

Jim terminated his child analysis 5 days before his twelfth birthday. Although I thought of him many times in the intervening years, there was no direct contact until I greeted him 13 years later at age 26, in the same office.

His mother had called once, when Jim was in high school, asking for a referral for a friend. When I asked how Jim was doing, the response was a sparse "fine."

Jim asked to see me, because he was having difficulty deciding on a choice of career. Greeting him in the waiting room was somewhat of a shock since I half expected to see the preadolescent boy I had come to know so well. In his stead was a handsome, slimly built young man, over 6 feet tall. The one clear link between the boy and the man was a distinctive broad smile.

Jim readily told me of his occupational doubts. He loved golf and wanted to make a career as a professional golfer but was concerned about the financial uncertainty of such a venture. He had graduated from a major university 2 years ago and was living at home, working occasionally and contending with his parents' dissatisfaction with his life. A second problem of significance emerged as Jim began to describe his adolescent and adult development. A summary of that information, which was gathered over the subsequent year-and-one half, follows.

The junior high school years were good ones. Jim went through puberty easily between 13 and 14, had many friends, and was very active in sports. He easily maintained a B+ to A– average throughout high school and college. The always difficult relationship with his father improved considerably during adolescence because of Jim's academic and athletic success and his plans to attend college. However, Jim and his father were never close and were at loggerheads again because the father was dissatisfied with Jim's lack of direction.

During adolescence Jim had not been a disciplinary problem at home or in school and had never been involved with the police. Jim had intercourse for the first time at the end of the tenth grade and dated fairly regularly throughout high school and college, but, significantly, had only one steady girlfriend during those years. He did not currently have a girlfriend and was not looking for one since he doubted that he would ever marry. Occasional, casual contacts were easy to come by and met his sexual needs.

Toward the middle of our first session, Jim volunteered that he began smoking pot off and on in high school and smoked "a lot" in college. "I still do," he continued, "three to four times per week . . . it makes me happy with the status quo." If he were me, he continued, he would tell himself to stop smoking pot, and to give up alcohol, which he also used several times per week.

After several visits, I conveyed my concern about the significance of Jim's drug use and offered various ways to address it. Jim decided to try to stop on his own and asked if I would agree to see him 2 or 3 times a month. When I suggested that more frequent visits would be necessary because of the severity of his problems, he calmly stood his ground. After expressing doubts about his plan, but in the face of his determination to do it his way—he had not lost his strength of conviction since his analysis—I agreed to see him as often as he wished for a trial period.

To my surprise he did make dramatic change in his life, including stopping drinking and smoking pot—cold turkey!

Within a month, Jim got a job as a clerk at a large discount chain. The boring, routine work, which he saw as an indicator of what was ahead if he did not change, served as a stimulus to begin addressing the issue of his future. As we discussed various possibilities, Jim returned again and again to his wish to become a high school teacher. In order to test out his interest, he spent 6 highly enjoyable months as an unpaid teacher's aide and then enrolled in a full-time program, while maintaining his job, which will provide him with a teaching credential in the near future. The increase in self-esteem was almost palpable as his wish to become a teacher—highly valued by himself and his parents—began to become a reality.

I could see two other major dynamic conflicts which would impede Jim's young adult development in the near future, neither of which was likely to be resolved as easily as the drug dependence and choice of career. They are his unresolved, Oedipally-based conflicts with his father, which are interfering with the third individuation and his fear of intimacy, marriage, and parenthood, also the result of neurotic conflict and inhibition. As I understand it, the central dynamic issue is the same one which was present during the child analysis—rage at the Oedipal father, who is still experienced as distant and disapproving in real life, but even more importantly, is firmly internalized in the superego and ego ideal.

As a result of our work during the child analysis, enough modification occurred in the superego to allow adolescent development to occur fairly uneventfully. Jim was able to achieve enough academically, socially, and athletically to bolster his self-esteem and satisfy his own and his father's expectations.

This intrapsychic state of affairs continued throughout high school and college but collapsed when Jim left the protected environment of academia where, because of his intelligence, he was easily able to achieve what was expected of him by his superego and his parents—to maintain a respectable grade point average and graduate. When he entered young adulthood and was unable to successfully engage the first developmental task that confronted him, namely, the transition to either graduate school or the adult working world, he became anxious and depressed and resorted to drug and alcohol use in order to "be happy with the status quo."

Jim did not continue to think analytically on his own during adolescence. He had a developmental need to separate from me—as from his parents—in order to facilitate the second individuation. To have done so, to use his word, would have been "abnormal." This attitude is consistent with my experience with other adolescent patients. It was only when Jim began to develop symptoms in his early twenties that thoughts about me and our work together began to "intrude" into his consciousness.

I think these observations illustrate the power and the limitations of therapy in childhood to resolve conflicts and influence the course of subsequent development. When Jim began analysis, he was an unhappy, isolated latency-aged boy. As a result of our efforts, he was able to engage the difficult developmental issues of adolescence with relative ease.

But clearly, our work together did not sufficiently resolve his Oedipal conflicts with his father to allow him to successfully make the transition to young adulthood. Perhaps I am expecting too much of both of us since the goal of treatment is to allow the patient to return to the developmental mainstream and not to promise to ensure him or her against the vicissitudes of life or new developmental demands.

John

Now let us turn our attention to John L. who entered therapy at age 38. John L. presented himself as a trim, well-dressed man with streaks of gray in his hair. He was self-referred because, despite a happy marriage and a successful law practice, he was increasingly anxious to the point of panic and had been experiencing fleeting thoughts of running away. John L. had little idea what was upsetting him but knew it was "time to talk to somebody."

John L. had married for the second time 5 years ago to a woman who had 2 sons, currently aged 12 and 14. He had a 15-year-old son of his own from his first marriage who lived with his mother in a nearby city. John L.'s own mother was dead but his father was alive and well.

Initially John L. attributed his symptoms primarily to work. His solo practice, in a city overflowing with lawyers, was very successful but demanded 80+ hours per week of his time. Good help was difficult to find and keep, and it seemed as though his entire existence revolved around his law practice. His wife thought he worked entirely too hard but demanded little of his time or energy until recently when her 14-year-old son began to manifest behavioral problems at home and in school. John L. did what he could to help but felt increasingly guilty as he spent more and more time with his stepson and even less with his natural son, whom he saw only sporadically at best.

The mention of his natural son was accompanied by a striking increase in free-floating anxiety and an unrecognized revelation of important conflictual material. John L.'s girlfriend had become pregnant with his son when they were college students. Both of them had been virgins prior to dating each other and had only engaged in intercourse three or four times when the pregnancy occurred. His parents were dismayed by the pregnancy since they did not like his girlfriend and wanted John L. to complete his education before marrying.

When John L.'s father announced that he would no longer pay for his son's college education, John L. said one word "Oh?" and left. The two men never discussed the matter again. John L. did marry his girl-friend and was cut off financially. He, in turn, withdrew emotionally. In the past 20 years, contact with his parents had consisted of four or five frosty phone conversations initiated by his mother and a false display of family togetherness at her funeral 5 years ago.

The marriage was difficult from the start, beginning as it did with a pregnancy and an absence of family blessing or financial resources. John L. did manage to stay in college—his wife dropped out to care for the baby—but within a short period of time he knew that the marriage was a mistake. He loved his young son desperately but was increasingly distant from his wife who seemed "superficial, boring and fat." After graduation and a brief trial of marriage counseling, he took off for California, feeling "exhilarated and free—I finally had all of it off my back."

After working for a while John L. put himself through law school. His former wife followed him, hoping for a reconciliation, but to no avail. She eventually married a man who made little money but was a decent stepfather. John L. was painfully aware of the difference between the very comfortable life-style which he provided for his two stepchildren and the rather meager circumstances under which his natural son lived.

When John L. met his second wife, he felt exhilarated and happy for the first time in many years. She was outgoing, uninhibited sexually and, "made me the center of her life." They were married within 6 months. His new stepsons, quiet and unassuming latency-aged boys, "seemed like nice kids, I didn't give them much thought."

Developmental History. John L. did not remember much about his early years but gradually a picture emerged of a quiet, somewhat shy child who was physically healthy and who did not manifest any obvious psychological problems or developmental delays or deviations. His mother was at home on a full-time basis and seemed to enjoy raising her son.

John L.'s memories of latency were clear and not particularly happy. Although an excellent student, he was small in stature and frequently teased. He had a few friends but felt "on the outside looking in." His father pushed him into sports where he did not excel, and seemed disappointed in him.

Puberty occurred late, in tenth grade. "I remember erections, wet dreams, and thoughts about girls." When I commented on the absence of masturbation from his list, John L. blushed and said, "that was so good I knew it must be terrible in some way."

College was a time of greater acceptance socially, a sense of "liberation" from his father, and the beginning of dating and a sexual life.

Unfortunately, this heady sense of exhilaration and freedom was short-lived, quickly replaced by premature work, marriage, and parenthood.

I made a diagnosis of anxiety neurosis and presented a recommendation for therapy. After a discussion about schedule and finances, John L. agreed to begin twice-weekly psychotherapy. Because of the focus of this chapter, I will address the clinical material which relates to our consideration of development in young adulthood.

John L.'s sexual inhibitions emerged as a central theme in the treatment fairly early on. As we analyzed his masturbation, strongly repressed phallic and exhibitionistic fantasies emerged. For example, he pictured himself as an Arab sheik lounging on silk pillows in a richly decorated palace, choosing his sexual companion for the night from his harem girls who paraded suggestively before him. As he anticipated the sexual adventure ahead, his erection began to grow, and grow, and grow, breaking through the ceiling and continuing skyward, not unlike Jack's beanstalk. The gradual disappearance of John L.'s sexual inhibitions led to a return of his masturbation and an enhanced sex life with his wife.

The analysis of the transference, specifically the interpretation of John L.'s great concern about my reaction to his phallic aggressiveness, led to many associations about his father. Gradually he tested my ability to accept his rage at the father/therapist, eventually spewing forth blast after blast at his father for his coldness and insensitivity, particularly in regard to the pregnancy. Signs of softening and wishes for reconciliation followed, stimulated by our work, to be sure, but also propelled by the patient's position on the threshold of midlife. As he approached the age of 40 and his father 70, he became increasingly aware that if a reconciliation were to take place, it better occur soon, and it did. John L. called his father, who was mildly receptive, and eventually went, along with his son, to visit him. John L. was surprised at the pleasure and degree of inner comfort which he experienced during the visit but was totally unprepared—and consciously jealous of—the warmth of the rapport which developed almost instantly between the grandfather and the grandson; for they, too, were strangers just getting to know each other. John L. and his father have continued to develop their relationship which is beginning to take the form of a reversal of generations as John increasingly cares for his aging father—not without a sense of superiority for being there for his father in his time of need.

In the months following the rapprochement between the son and the father, John L.'s associations increasingly turned to his relationship with his own son. Following the acceptance of the painful interpretation that he had abandoned his son just as his father had abandoned him, John L. increased their contact and eventually invited his son to come and live with him, "during the few years that are left before he becomes a man." The transition took place after several months of patient negotiation with both wives.

Watching John L.'s guilt diminish and self-esteem grow as he incorporated the role of full-time father was a rewarding experience for patient and therapist alike. Although personally satisfying, detailed contact with his son also led to the realization that the teenager was struggling, primarily with social relationships. In a bittersweet burst of newly found similarity, John L. recognized that, "he looks like me, is beginning to talk like me—and seems to have the same problems I did. At least he'll get help when he's 15, not 40."

His wife's kindness to his son surprised him and precipitated more guilt since John L. had accepted her children but not the role of their stepfather. Gradually he came to accept the realization that he had three teenaged sons to raise and support.

The development of his relationship with the three boys and his father as well as the more intimate, less inhibited relationship with his wife filled John L. with a sense of integrity and competence that he had never experienced before. "For the first time in life I'm doing what I ought to be doing—I'm being a good husband, father, and son. I wish my Mom were alive to see this. I think she'd be very proud of me."

But the joy and pleasure in these relationships, the shift from a life almost devoid of closeness to one overflowing with intensity, led to the realization that John L. was responsible for his loved ones. Increasingly, he began to recognize and accept that as an involved midlife husband, father, and son he had assumed the "burden" of caring for his father as he aged and eventually died, of raising his sons, including the probability of putting all three of them through college, and of remaining emotionally and sexually intimate with his wife in a sustained relationship. "It's tough," he said, "but it's great. Life does begin at 40!"

CONSIDERATION OF THE CLINICAL MATERIAL FROM A DEVELOPMENTAL STANDPOINT

The usefulness of adult developmental concepts for the clinician is demonstrated both by the manner of presentation of the case material and the discussion of it in relationship to some of the young adult developmental tasks which were presented earlier in the chapter.

The Third Individuation. As previously described, the transition from the second to the third individuation is a young adult experience, stimulated by the growing capacity for intrapsychic separation from the parents and engagement of the phase-specific developmental tasks of young adulthood. This normative process was partially arrested in both Jim and John L.; consequently, neither functioned as emotionally self-sufficient individuals in their 20s. Jim's libidinal and aggressive drives remain primarily focused on his parents. Many interpretive interventions addressed the degree to which Jim continued to seek his parents' approval for his young adult aspirations and actions, indicated by the degree of rage he experienced when that approval was withheld.

John L., on the other hand, was individuating rather easily—as evidenced by the growing sense of emotional self-sufficiency at college, academic success, and the beginning of an adult sexual pattern—until the unexpected pregnancy and his parents' reaction to it arrested the process. Although John L. appeared to have mastered the third individuation—he married, became a father, had a successful career, and moved to another state—in reality he repressed his primarily neurotic conflicts around sexuality and aggression, and ran away from his wife, son, and parents. This state of affairs continued until the death of his mother, the approaching old age of his father, and the adolescence of his son upset the tenuous emotional equilibrium which had existed through much of his young adulthood and resulted in the outbreak of an anxiety neurosis. The unconscious command was do something about these relationships before time runs out!

Developing the Capacity for Intimacy. The emergence of the capacity for intimacy in early young adulthood was compromised in both Jim and John L. Because Jim's identification with his father was so conflicted, he was still strongly rejecting the idea of becoming a lover and a husband. Based on his child analysis, I can also propose that at an unconscious level he had not sufficiently abandoned the Oedipal wish to possess his mother and become involved in an intimate relationship with another. However, as therapy progressed, Jim began to acknowledge his avoidance and to explore the inhibition, eventually becoming involved in a loving relationship with a woman and considering marriage, although this relationship eventually ended because of a mutual preoccupation with career advancement. Jim is now able to openly acknowledge his desire for intimacy and children.

John L. married his first wife out of need and spite. As their relationship was compromised by pregnancy, parenthood, and near poverty, he emotionally withdrew from her. It took more than 10 years before he allowed himself to become emotionally involved with another woman. For a second time, he began to fuse sexual and loving feelings, this time in an environment far removed from parental influence and with a woman much more advanced than he along the developmental line of the capacity for intimacy. In fact, some of the anxiety which precipitated the search for treatment was related to a growing conscious awareness that he could not match his wife's level of sexual freedom and comfort or her desire for emotional closeness. The removal of many of his sexual inhibitions through treatment made it possible for him to sustain an intimate relationship with a woman for the first time in his life. To quote him, "life does begin at forty."

Becoming a Father. The experience of impregnating a woman adds a new dimension to a young man's sexual identity by confirming that his penis and testicles are capable of performing the primary function for which they are intended. For most males in their teens and early twenties, the goal is avoidance of this state. When an active, purposeful attempt is made to become a father, a powerful psychological process is begun. One newly married man described the conscious aspect of the process as follows: "I've always enjoyed sex, but now that my wife and I are trying to have a baby it's totally different. I hope we can do it. It will be pretty awful if we can't."

Jim's most scathing criticism of his father was and is reserved for his performance as a father. Since I had contact with his father during the child analysis, I know that there was a considerable amount of distortion in Jim's evaluation even though his father did have very high standards for himself and his son and was somewhat distant. Regardless of the cause, Jim's current problem was that he saw fatherhood as a burden, a source of pain and conflict; not as one of young adulthood's richest experiences which will fulfill developmental potential along several different lines. As he analyzed his feelings of inferiority about himself as a young adult (particularly the need to live at home and receive financial support) and anticipated the day in the not too distant future when he would be financially independent and involved in a career which had a great social value in both his and his father's eyes, Jim's feelings about parenthood began to change. Gradually, he came to accept the fact that his father had done the best job that he could—and that Jim would do a better one with his children.

Unlike Jim, John L. became a biological father in his early twenties but avoided a psychological commitment to his son for over 10 years. Like Jim, his failure to become a committed psychological parent was based on his conflicted identification with his father. He attempted to master the devastating psychological abandonment by his father when his girlfriend became pregnant by doing to his son what was done to him. But again like Jim, there was a strong positive aspect to this relationship with his father which facilitated his masculine development during childhood and became internalized in his superego and ego ideal. Thus, he could not rid himself of the internalized father, or the internalized son. Eventually, without conscious awareness, he had to seek help to rid himself of his guilt by analyzing his conflicts about the roles of father and son relationships and then reestablish his ties with the two most important men in his life while there was still time to effect their adolescent and late-life development.

Developing a Relationship of Mutuality and Equality with Parents while facilitating Their Mid- and Late-Life Development. Jim is a long way from establishing a sense of mutuality and equality with his father, but it will likely happen as he becomes a teacher, achieves financial independence, marries, and has a family; in other words, when he masters the major developmental tasks of young adulthood. It is hoped, for both him and his father, that he will facilitate his father's mid- and late-life development by providing him with grandchildren, and that when the time comes, he will take care of his father during his declining years.

As John L. nears forty, he is deeply engaged in this process with his father. His reward is a deep inner sense of integrity and authority, and for the first time in many years, the absence of guilt.

When their normal development is not significantly impeded adolescent males enter young adulthood, that marvelous time of life when masculinity reaches mature fruition; and in the process they become independent adults, loving husbands, and last but not least, fathers to their sons and eventually fathers to their fathers. A more detailed consideration of the treatment of these two men may be found in "Traversing Young Adulthood, The Male Journey from Twenty to Forty" in the *Psychoanalytic Inquiry* (Colarusso, in press).

TRANSITION TO MIDLIFE

Levinson *et al.* (1978) described early adulthood (ages 17–45) as ending with a period that he called the *midlife transition* (between 40 and 45). The concept of transition from early to middle adulthood is valid, although the chronology may not be as precise as Levinson indicates. The evidence for active, dynamic psychological development in midlife is growing (Levinson *et al.*, 1978; Vaillant, 1990; Eichorn, Clausen & Haan, 1981) as is the recognition of both thematic continuity and clear distinctions between the two developmental phases.

The shift toward middle adulthood is driven by powerful biological and psychological forces, such as the aging process in the body, the growth of children into adolescence and young adulthood, work achievement or failure, and the aging, illness, and death of parents (Nemiroff & Colarusso, 1985).

Because of these internal and external pressures the major intrapsychic issues of young adulthood—intimacy, procreation, and achievement—are gradually replaced by:

1. A shift from thinking of oneself as young to thinking of oneself as old (Neugarten, 1979).
2. A new sense of self—shaped by the recognition of advancing age and personal time limitation; urgent searching for ways to gratify the self and define priorities while there is still time.
3. A desire to leave a meaningful legacy after death—to have made an impact on the world, to be remembered.
4. The maintenance of sexual intimacy in the face of diminished sexual urgency and the aging body (Gould, 1978). Critical assessment of the marriage(s) in regard to success or failure and reexamination of the commitment to continue in the relationship or seek a new one before time runs out (Berrman & Lief, 1975).
5. The acceptance of grown children and their family members as independent beings of great value to the mid- and late-life development of the parents.
6. Completion of the shift from protégé to mentor.

CHAPTER 11

Middle Adulthood (Ages 40–60)

INTRODUCTION

Recently, Roger Gould (1990) said "concepts of time, aging, and death represent the 'entities' of the life-cycle developmental process. Therapeutic attention can no longer focus entirely on the conflicts of memory; it must include current reality and the struggle to adapt to ever-changing time" (p. 346). Certainly, these issues are at the core of understanding and treating individuals between the ages of 40 and 60, that is, those who are in *midlife*. Despite the ominous sound of time, aging, and death, the middle years are probably the best time in life for many. Middle adulthood is the golden age of adulthood (similar to late latency in childhood, although much longer) because it is an interval of relative stability characterized (for most) by physical health, emotional maturity, a clearly defined sense of self, competence and power in the work situation, and gratifying relationships with spouse, children, parents, friends, and colleagues.

THE TRANSITION FROM YOUNG TO MIDDLE ADULTHOOD

There is no sharp physical or psychological demarcation between young and middle adulthood. The process of physical retrogression, begun in young adulthood, picks up speed and becomes a powerful organizing influence on intrapsychic life; but the change is slow, unlike for example, the sudden biological upheaval of puberty which initiates the adolescent process. Psychologically, midlife is a time of significant change—the mind of the 50-year-old is qualitatively different from that of the 30-year-old—but, as with the aging process in the body, the transformation is gradual and not experienced as a disruption.

Stevens-Long (1990) described the transition in social terminology.

> Development in young adulthood seems to be embedded in close relationships. Intimacy, love, commitment, and the analysis of relationships within a finite system—all seem related to the mastery of those relationships most immediate to personal experience. The transition from young adulthood to middle age implies a widening of concern to the larger social system. The emergence of intrasystemic thinking implies the differentiation of one's own social, political, and historical system from others, appreciation of its strengths and weaknesses, and an ability to identify with, and hence feel compassion for, another human system. In young adulthood we learn to comprehend and identify with another human system. (p. 154)

Erikson (1963) described middle adulthood in terms of generativity, Maslow (1968) spoke of self-actualization, Jung (1933) and Edelstein and Noam (1982) of wisdom. I will incorporate these ideas and those of other theoreticians under the discussion of the developmental tasks of midlife.

THE DEVELOPMENTAL TASKS
OF MIDDLE ADULTHOOD

Accepting the Aging Process in the Body

As described in Chapter Ten on young adulthood, physical decline begins to have an effect on psychological development in the 20s and 30s. However, by the 40s and 50s, because of the extremely obvious, universal evidence of physical retrogression and the marked increase in major illnesses and the death of contemporaries, thoughts and feelings about the aging body become a major, sometimes dominant influence, on mental life. Marcia Goin (1990) described the effect as follows:

> *The appearance of one's body in midlife takes on a different significance.* Efforts to remain trim and fit are not made to develop a sense of identity or to separate and individuate, but to maintain health and youthfulness and to deter the effects of aging. The struggle is to retain body integrity in the face of anxieties about aging, the vulnerabilities of failing health, and the potential loss of independence. (p. 524)

In addition to the obvious differences in vision, hair color, reflexes, and skin tone, there are equally important changes in the more private aspects of physical functioning. These include cessation of menstruation, increase in urinary frequency and diminished force of the urinary stream, and alterations in sexual functioning. These will be considered under the developmental line of intimacy, love, and sex.

The response to these dramatic biological changes varies enormously from individual to individual, as evidenced by the myriad "symptoms" which are related to the menopause. Recent research (Eisdorfer & Raskind, 1975) has determined that the emotional lability, depression, irritability, and increased somatic complaints are individual psychological responses which are present to varying degrees in a minority of women. Only the cessation of menses and hot flashes are directly related to the decreased production of estrogen.

Each midlife individual must engage the developmental task of *mourning for the lost body of youth*. The physical changes just described are experienced mentally in the form of body monitoring—a continual, conscious and unconscious, narcissistically injurious comparison of the midlife body with the body of childhood, adolescence, and young adulthood. This painful process leads to a *normative conflict* between wishes to deny the aging process and acceptance of the loss of a youthful body (Colarusso & Nemiroff, 1981). Pathological attempts to deny aging include uses of plastic surgery; attempts at fusion with younger bodies; inappropriate physical competition with younger individuals; the acquisition of possessions, such as art, automobiles, or clothing which become narcissistically gratifying substitutes for the body; and failure to care for the body through the avoidance of regular checkups, exercise, and a healthy diet.

A more normative "resolution" (there is no actual resolution since the process continues for the rest of life) leads to a major change in the body image which gradually comes to include a more realistic, less painful picture of the body and the ability to enjoy the pleasures which the midlife body can continue to provide, particularly if it is cared for properly.

The Acceptance of Time Limitation and Personal Death

Stimulated by both biology and the environment, by the aging process in the body, and by such experiences as the death of parents and contemporaries, the growth of children into adulthood, and grandparenthood and the approach of retirement, the individual in this developmental phase comes face-to-face with his or her mortality with the painful, but unavoidable recognition that the future is limited and that he or she will die.

Thoughts and feelings about having a limited amount of time left to live increase in frequency and intensity and become an extremely powerful organizer, forcing a significant reexamination of all aspects of how life has been lived in the past; its present positive and negative aspects, particularly in regard to marriage, family, and work; and a reassessment of how to use the time that is left.

The increased preoccupation with aging and time limitation leads to what Jung (1933) called *midlife introversion* and Neugarten called (1979) *interiority*. The increasing preoccupation with the meaning of life, the assessment of personal successes and failures, the intense scrutiny of interpersonal relationships, and the lessened interest in new challenges are the midlife equivalent of the life review (Butler and Lewis, 1977) which is such a central aspect of late life development.

Cohler and Lieberman (1979) and Lieberman and Tobin (1983) have conducted studies which indicate that persons in their 40s and 50s experience increased concern about health, lowered self-esteem, anxiety, and depression. These symptoms are indicative of the intense developmental process which is going on, leading to what Levinson *et al.* (1978) called the *midlife transition* (normative) or to the onset, sometimes for the first time, of psychiatric illness (Guttman, Griffin, & Grunes, 1982).

Gender-related differences in the expression of interiority have been demonstrated cross-culturally by Guttman (1977, 1987). He discovered that men become more passive and interested in being taken care of while becoming less involved in active mastery at home and at work. In contrast, women become more assertive, less interested in caring for their families, and increasingly directed toward activities beyond home and family (Back, 1974).

> As a consequence of increased awareness of the finitude of life, both men and women intensify concerns with self and display less patience for demands upon time and energy which are actively experienced as being in 'short supply' .... Realization of goals and reworking the presently understood story of one's life course in order to maintain a sense of personal coherence become particularly important in late middle age and require time and energy, which is then less available for other pursuits. (Cohler & Galatzer-Levy, 1990, p. 226)

For others the mental work is primarily performed at an unconscious level. These individuals usually deny that time limitation or personal death occupy an important place in their mental life, but they demonstrate the same changes, normative or pathological, as their more aware counterparts.

The acceptance of personal time limitation can greatly enhance the quality of life for the healthy individual by stimulating an assessment of goals, a reordering of priorities, and a greater appreciation of significant relationships and the true value of time. For those individuals who come to midlife with significant pathology or a great sense of disappointment with life, attempting to accept this mortality may precipitate various forms of symptomatology or frantic actions, including the stereotypical—but very real—*midlife crisis* (to be discussed later in this chapter).

Acceptance of time limitation and personal death is a prerequisite for the engagement in late adulthood of the concern with *how* death will come, not if or when.

Intimacy, Love, and Sex—Maintaining Intimacy

Whereas the young adult is involved in developing the capacity for intimacy, the middle-aged person is focused on *maintaining* it in the face of powerful physical, psychological, and environmental pressures. In a long-standing relationship, inhibitors of sustaining physical and emotional closeness include changes in attitudes about sex and sexual functioning because of aging; psychological unavailability because of preoccupation with developmental pressures, such as the acceptance of time limitation and personal death; and the realistic demands of work and provisions for children and elderly parents.

In newer relationships which begin in midlife, all of the above factors may operate, sometimes multiplied by a factor of two or more. In addition other issues, unique to second beginnings, such as the absence of a history together and a network of longstanding friendships; age and generational differences between the partners, for example, in regard to having children; or the problems of constituting a step family may interfere with the development and maintenance of intimacy.

In regard to sexual functioning, the task is twofold: (1) to accept the appearance of the middle-aged body and continue to find it sexually stimulating and (2) to accept changes in the ability of the body to perform sexually. For some individuals, the partner's body remains sexually stimulating or diminished interest is compensated for by feelings of love and tenderness generated over the years by a satisfying relationship. Others who cannot accept the change in the partner's body stop having sex, have affairs, or leave the marriage, usually in search of a younger person.

Normative changes in sexual functioning, which increase in frequency and intensity as this phase of development progresses, include diminished sexual drive and ability to perform mechanically. Men have more difficulty achieving and sustaining erections and may experience a longer refractory period after ejaculation. Because of diminished estrogen production, women experience a thinning of the vaginal mucosa, a decrease in the rate and amount of lubrication, and a small decrease in the number of contractions at the time of orgasm (Masters & Johnson, 1966).

These physical changes produce powerful psychological responses, normative and pathological, which affect every patient in this age group. Because the subject matter is embarrassing for some and painful for others, many patients will avoid this area entirely and resist attempts by the therapist to introduce the subject of sexual functioning and emotional intimacy.

Environmental interferences with the task of maintaining intimacy are usually considerable during midlife. The demands of raising children, either adolescents in a first marriage or younger stepchildren in a second one, interfere with the privacy and emotional equilibrium required for intimacy as do the pressures and responsibilities of work. Fatigue and diminished interest are common denominators in these circumstances. Individuals with more deeply rooted problems with sexuality or relationships will use the aging process or the preoccupation with work, children, or elderly parents to rationalize their conflicts and avoid analyzing them.

As part of the reappraisal, both partners experience intense feelings of nostalgia for former lovers, mourn for missed opportunities, and struggle with the question of whether to settle for the status quo or fling themselves into the jungle of the middle-aged singles world in search of greater perfection. For many, the conflict rages internally. For others, it is accompanied by action in the form of affairs, trial separations, and divorce.

Divorce has great consequences not only for the two individuals involved but also for their loved ones. The ripple effect can have major consequences for children, parents, friends, and colleagues. Sometimes, because of unrecognized and untreated psychopathology, the divorced individual fails to find a more satisfying relationship or repeats ingrained patterns. However, other divorced individuals are able to establish a new relationship in which the quest for a richer sexual and emotional relationship is realized.

CLINICAL EXAMPLES

Various forms of therapeutic intervention, such as marital counseling, individual psychotherapy, and psychoanalysis, can be extremely effective in helping individuals decide what to do or deal with the consequences of their partner's actions. Problems relating to intimacy, love, and sex occupy a prominent place in an outpatient practice. All four of the following examples were part of my practice at the same time.

Fifty-five-year-old Mrs. A. requested treatment "in order to leave my marriage. We've been married for 35 years but I haven't loved my husband for the last 20. I've been so dependent on him all of my adult life that I don't know if I have the courage to leave." During the course of twice-weekly psychotherapy which lasted 15 months, Mrs. A. left her husband, started her own business, and began a new relationship. "I have less money and I'm scared about the future, but I feel alive and in control of my life. I think Bill is happier, too."

Mr. S.'s marriage was a continuous preoccupation during his four-year analysis which began when he was 43. Very inhibited sexually during adolescence, he "married the only girl in the world who knew less about sex than I did." Twenty-three years, two children, and one affair later, he eventually decided to stay in the marriage. "I've learned in this analysis that sex is not the rare, extraordinary thing I thought it was as a kid; billions of people do it every day. I know I could go out and sleep with a lot of different women, but how different, or better, would it actually be? Jane and I have built a pretty good life together. She's changed a lot and so have I. I think we can make the next 20 years better than the last 20."

Mr. V. nearly fell apart when his wife of 21 years left him for another man. For 2 years, our weekly psychotherapy sessions focused on his shock, depression, and anger. At age 52 he found dating strange but was soon sleeping with many different women in a compulsive attempt to reassure himself about his deeply damaged sense of masculine competence. Repeated interpretation diminished the pattern but 4 years after the divorce he was still unable "to take a chance on getting that close to a woman again."

Mrs. T. left her "wonderful" husband because "I've missed something. I just have to get out on my own." Now 60, but married at age 18, she recognized that her rage at her husband for "not being all the other men I could have married, for closing off all the living I could have done" was irrational but uncontrollable. Now 6 months into the separation she has decided to live on her own "for a while" but fully intends to return to her husband. As we explore the infantile and adult issues which precipitated her leaving, the future of the marriage remains in doubt.

RELATIONSHIP TO CHILDREN—LETTING GO, ACHIEVING EQUALITY, AND INTEGRATING NEW FAMILY MEMBERS

Middle adulthood is the phase of development in which one's children become adolescents and young adults. Their inevitable progression through the phases of childhood, adolescence, and young adulthood affects every aspect of the parent's life. The manner in which the once all powerful progenitors let go of their children, their work to achieve a new relationship with them, which is based on equality and mutuality, and to integrate in-laws and grandchildren into their lives can make the difference between a life full of richness and love or one rampant with rancor, bitterness, and emptiness.

Letting Go

Young adult parental vigor and the (it is hoped positive and facilitating) unchallenged control of young children go hand in hand; but so do the middle-age awareness of physical decline and time limitation and the inevitable loss of control of adolescent and young adult offspring. The transition from the first to the second state was vividly described by Gerald Pearson (1958):

> by the time an individual is in his late thirties or early forties—usually when his children are becoming adolescents—he begins to realize that he will never fulfill some of his postponed ideals. He perceives that he has already started on the down grade toward old age and death, and this realization invigorates his fantasy of the reversal of generations (p. 177) . . . he observes that his adolescent child is growing rapidly into a vigorous young adult with all his success ahead of him. He contrasts his lessening opportunities for success and his now rather static capacities with the budding development of his child, and unconsciously he feels envy. In his unconscious his child now seems to be a replica of his own parent; and he begins to act to keep the child in his place just as he wanted to put his parents in his place when he was a child. (p. 21)

Although the feelings described by Pearson are experienced by every parent, healthy ones do not consistently act on them; instead they gradually relinquish control over their children's lives, experiencing in the process feelings of weakness, passivity, and rage. Because some of the pleasure of parenting is related to the direct and sublimated expression of aggression through control of the child, the loss of such power is painful (Colarusso & Nemiroff, 1982).

For many parents and children the gradual shift in the balance of power between them, which takes place over many adolescent and young adult years, is symbolized by a single event which has been described by Nemiroff and myself as "the moment of truth," referring to the climatic moment in the corrida when the matador kills the bull (Nemiroff & Colarusso, 1985). Many middle-aged patients (and therapists) can describe that moment in time in which they knew that their "child" had gained the upper hand. The "moment" may be physical or psychological as exemplified by being playfully pinned against the wall by a son or daughter—and being unable to break free; or losing a game of bowling or a tennis match when you have tried as hard as you could; or being outshouted in a battle over the Saturday-night curfew and realizing that your teenager would be home closer to his or her chosen hour than yours.

Facilitating the developing sexuality of adolescent children is also a difficult task for the middle-aged parent because of the juxtaposition between his or her waning sexuality and the adolescent's sexual promise. In addition, more liberal sexual attitudes and mores often add to the parent's discomfort by making the contrast between the parent's experience and the adolescent's opportunities quite distinct, particularly for women. The healthy parent struggles with these conscious and unconscious concerns but gradually accepts the fact that sons and daughters are likely to begin dating in midadolescence and become sexually active in late adolescence.

Conscious concerns about their children's burgeoning sexuality and the reactivation of unresolved sexual conflicts from their childhood and adult past are often presenting themes in the treatment of middle-aged patients. For others, this area is a source of great resistance because of conscious embarrassment over excessive interest in, or undue restriction of, the adolescent's sexual development, and the arousal of unconscious incestuous feelings. The therapist who has a fundamental knowledge of child and adult development is better able to help the patient deal with the interplay of infantile, adolescent, and adult sexual issues which are the determinants behind the patient's symptomatology and his or her interaction with their sons and daughters.

Each developmental transition brings with it the prospect of significant change in the balance and equilibrium which previously existed intrapsychically and in relationships. David Guttman (1990), the cultural anthropologist, suggested that biological retrogression and the disappearance of the parental function produce a radical change in the individual psyches of mothers and fathers and in their relationship.

> My studies of older men and women in various cultures have led to this conclusion: late development and late-onset pathology are often fueled by the same forces. They are driven by energies, released in men and women, in the course of the postparental transition toward androgeny ... the gender distinctions, which emerge most sharply when young parents enter what I have termed *the chronic emergency* of parenthood, get blurred as the last children are launched, usually in the parents' middle years ... postparental men appropriate qualities of nurturance and tenderness that were once relatively alien within themselves, and only tolerable in their dependents—their wives or children. By the same token, postparental women adopt some of the ascendant, competitive qualities that their husbands are relinquishing. As each postparental spouse becomes as the other used to be, the couple moves toward the

normal androgeny of later life. Given its linkage to the genetic requirements of parenthood, the so-called contrasexual transition is, like paternity and maternity themselves, a quasi-universal event. As such, it usually precedes a developmental advance. Indeed, after some period of psychic dislocation, most men and women do accommodate to the changes in themselves and in their spouses. They gradually craft the energies liberated by the postparental reversal into new executive capacities of the personality. They do not at the same time lose their gender identities as men or women: instead, they revise their self-conception to include the new powers that accompany the midlife transformation. The result, for most men and women, is an expanded sense of self rather than a loss of self-continuity. The contrasexual upheavals of the postparental period have brought about new constancies in the form of new structures, new ego capacities for knowing and enjoying: psychological development has taken place. (pp. 171–172)

But the relationship between parents and their grown children has not ended, it has the potential to be transformed into something qualitatively different from what existed before—and just as gratifying. Such an outcome requires the concerted effort of both the young adult "child" and the middle-aged parent as they attempt to structure a new equality, a new mutuality, a new relationship which is in many ways more complex than the one which existed when they were younger.

Achieving Equality

As the parent moves into the later stages of middle adulthood and the son or daughter into the second half of young adulthood, all vestiges of the "child" disappear. Physically, the youthful appearance of the adolescent and the adult of the early 20s is gradually replaced by the obviously mature young adult who may already show signs of aging. He or she is very likely living away from home, significantly involved with others sexually and emotionally, raising children, and supporting himself or herself. The presence of these adult relationships and capabilities pushes the healthy parent–child relationship toward equality but is not in and of itself evidence that the acceptance of the equality has been achieved by either the parent or the child.

For example, 25-year-old Ron complained bitterly in his therapy that his mother, aged 57, continued to treat him like a child. Indeed she did. On a recent visit home to attend a family wedding, the mother had insisted that Ron's slacks and sport coat were "inappropriate" for the occasion. When an argument ensued, Ron's father stepped in, as he had always done, and encouraged his son to change his clothes, which he did. Ron could readily recognize his parents' need to control and infantilize him but he was unaware of his own conflict over the wish to appease his mother so as to remain emotionally involved and dependent and the desire to be independent. Over the course of two years of psychotherapy, as he came to recognize his own issues and the fact that his parents had no control over him that he did not give them, Ron began to make more independent decisions. At first, the changes in Ron's behavior intensified his mother's attempts to control him. Then she gradually began to work through her feelings of rage, impotence, and loss of control and begrudgingly moved toward a more equal relationship.

The healthy parent not only accepts the "child's" desire for independence and autonomy but also facilitates moves in that direction whenever possible by, for example, applauding a job promotion, accepting a potential spouse, or contributing to the downpayment on a home.

The reasons for such behavior are not entirely altruistic; they are based, in part, on the recognition of the central importance of the child and his or her new family to the parent's mid and late life development.

Integrating New Members into the Family

Mother-in-law jokes are not merely the whimsical expression of some comic's humor, they are also reflections of a universal, developmental conflict between young adults and their middle-aged parents. The task for a middle-aged father and mother may be simply stated but difficult to achieve: Give up your position as the primary love object in your child's life to another, who will be experienced initially to some degree as a stranger and an interloper. Then accept the new partner as he or she is and work to cultivate his or her friendship. Once again, the underlying motivation is not selfless, but it is based on a desire to continue to occupy a central, although less important, role in the life of one's child, as well as a wish to form a relationship with a young adult who is hopefully interesting and enriching but who will also control to a large degree access to the child and the grandchildren.

Because the new partner and the parent of the same sex love the same person, a triangle, similar to the infantile Oedipal triangle, is created. This forces all three individuals to reengage and rework their infantile experience in this new adult context (Colarusso & Nemiroff, 1981). As with the infantile complex, the current rendition is only "resolved" gradually and partially, the outcome determined by the emotional intactness of the participants. The solution for the midlife parent may lie in the birth of grandchildren, those marvelous new beings who enrich life and provide a profound stimulus to mid- and late-life development by serving as a partial replacement for the "lost" child, reconnecting midlife development to childhood and offering the only mastery of death available—the opportunity to live on genetically through children and now grandchildren.

However, the attraction to grandchildren is not usually all consuming nor need it replace in importance or preference other interests. The failure of new parents to recognize that their parents have other interests than themselves and their children can be a source of conflict between the generations.

> Young adult daughters assume caregiving as an essential ingredient of family ties. However, many studies show grandparents rapidly become resentful of demands by their young adult offspring for assistance with babysitting . . . the daughter's reaction is sometimes a source of lowered morale for the middle-aged parent, who prefers "intimacy at a distance." (Cohler & Galatzer-Levy, 1990, p. 232)

RELATIONSHIP TO PARENTS—REVERSAL OF ROLES, DEATH, AND INDIVIDUATION

> The healthy adult recognizes, as part of his authentic appraisal of reality, the central position of change in his life. A basic aspect of that change is the shifting nature of significant emotional relationships. Adult involvement with loved ones such as children, parents, colleagues, and friends is in constant realignment. These ties continue to shift in middle age—when healthy marriages deepen in significance (while others break up on the shoals of middle-age developmental issues); parents die or become dependent; children grow and leave; and friends increase in importance and in some instances leave or die themselves. As opposed to old age and in some respects to childhood as well, the task is to sort out, categorize, set priorities among relationships, and achieve a balance between internal pressures and external demands. (Colarusso and Nemiroff, 1981, p. 90)

This basic change in the nature of relationships is particularly true of those between middle-aged children and their parents. At some point, as elderly parents become less able to care for themselves, a reversal of the roles in their lifelong relationships occurs. The "child" becomes the "parent" of the parent, increasingly fulfilling the roles of physical and mental caretaker.

A middle-aged patient described the change in her relationships with her 83-year-old mother. "It's sad. She used to be so vital. I remember her being so strong, when I was a child. She worked from day to night. Now I have to help her when she walks. Yesterday I had to cut her meat. I felt like I was taking care of a 2-year-old. But every once in a while she gets that spark back in her eyes and I remember what she was like for so many years. My daughter was there at the time. Neither one of us said anything, but I knew we were seeing ourselves in the same situation, 20 or 30 years in the future."

The relationship with her mother was a central aspect of this woman's therapy, stimulating both a reengagement of issues from the childhood and adolescent past and the consideration of phase-specific, current midlife themes.

Physical aging in the parents stimulates the ongoing intrapsychic process of psychological separation from them. The acute reversal of roles which occurs when parents are unable to take care of themselves forces the middle-aged child to anticipate the parent's demise.

Caring for aging parents is one of the most difficult—and most frequently avoided—developmental tasks in adulthood. In addition to presenting difficult realistic issues, such as arrangements for day-to-day care, it forces a reworking of childhood issues with the parents, engagement of the phase-specific, midlife acceptance of time limitation and personal death, and the anticipation of the inevitable role reversal which will occur with one's own children. Small wonder that the elderly are neglected and nursing homes are full. However, the avoidance of this developmental task has considerable psychological consequences, particularly guilt and depression. Clinicians who are aware of the enormous psychological power of this developmental process will pay close attention to their patient's associations in this area and will address the resistances to such material when it is absent.

Upon the death of an elderly parent, no matter how expected or unanticipated, a mourning process ensues. Long after the acute phase of this process is over the intrapsychic relationships with the dead parent continue to be dynamic and emotionally charged, an important subject for psychotherapeutic exploration.

In addition to stimulating thoughts about personal death, the demise of a parent also, almost paradoxically, stimulates thoughts and feelings about, and an interest in children and grandchildren. Besides partially filling the real and psychological void created by the death of parents, the relationships with children and grandchildren also facilitate the acceptance of time limitation and personal death by ensuring a form of psychological and genetic immortality, for it is they who will pass on the elder's genes and remember them when others forget.

FRIENDSHIPS

We are suggesting that because of the establishment of an adult sexual identity in the young adult years and because of the gratification gained from

adult sexual intimacy, mature midlife friendships (35–55) can be (but are not
necessarily) relatively desexualized compared to those that occur earlier in life.
(Nemiroff and Colarusso, 1985, p. 81)

The late adolescent's and the young adult's need to sexualize friendships and share sexual anxieties may be markedly diminished by the
mastery of sexuality and intimacy. Friendships with the opposite sex may
be easier to establish and maintain because needs for sexual satisfaction
and intimacy are being gratified elsewhere.

Midlife friendships do not usually have the sense of emotional intensity or the need for frequent physical presence of the friend, which are
characteristic of adolescence and to a lesser extent young adult relationships. This is because the healthy midlife individual has neither the
latency and adolescent need to build new psychic structure nor does the
pressing young adult need to find new friends and lovers.

Because of their unique position in the life cycle, men and women at
midlife can easily initiate and sustain friendships with individuals of
all ages. Unconscious motives underlie these relationships as they do
all others, but the midlife capacity for sublimation is considerable (Vaillant, 1977). The unconscious motivation behind friendships with adolescents and young adults may be the wish to identify with youth and an
abundant future as well the need to provide an outlet for sexual and
aggressive wishes related to parenthood and work. Friendships with
contemporaries may transparently reflect the increased awareness of old
age. For example, several couples decided to buy condominiums next to
each other to provide companionship and care in their old age. Successful
and independent in midlife, they had much in common in the present
and did not want to become dependent on their children in old age.

However, as at all other points in the life cycle, Freud's recognition
that friends can quickly become enemies or lovers remains completely
valid. Divorce, illness, retirement, or financial reversal can upset the
delicate balance of a friendship and alter its course, sometimes quickly
destroying relationships which have taken years to build.

WORK AND MENTORSHIPS:
THE EXERCISE OF POWER AND POSITION

For the majority of midlife adults in Western society, work is a
psychic organizer of major importance, regulating self-definition and
self-esteem, providing meaning and purpose to life, organizing the use of
time, and providing significant relationships and financial well-being.
Midlife in the work situation is the time of achievement and the exercise

of power, the result of years of effort during young and middle adulthood in which skills were mastered and seniority acquired.

The narcissistic gratifications related to work in midlife are often considerable, compensating for the painful realities of life relating to aging, parental death, and the loss of children. Sometimes the imbalance is such that work becomes the *main* source of emotional sustenance, resulting in a relative failure to engage the more difficult developmental issues of midlife and the neglect of vital relationships with spouse and children. Another result of an overinvestment in work may be an inability to recognize and plan for the eventual loss of work as a central organizing function; in other words, to plan for retirement and replacement by the next generation. The recognition of the juxtaposition of maximum achievement and power in the work place and the acceptance of loss and displacement is at the core of the midlife worker's intrapsychic life. Sometimes recognition of the conflict is facilitated by the phenomenon of *plateauing* (Bardwick, 1986): lateral movement in the workplace instead of promotion, indicating that the highest level of achievement possible has been attained.

Position in the work place includes the exercise of power toward subordinates, particularly younger ones who are potential successors. As one chief executive officer patient put it, "My toughest job is not running the company and making tough decisions, it's finding and training somebody to succeed me. I know whoever I choose will be grateful and appreciative, but they'll also be anxious to get me the hell out of there."

Contained therein is the essence of the conflict of the midlife mentor—to pass on knowledge and power to the next generation while recognizing that the mentee–mentor relationships are the means of one's displacement. In the healthy individual, the anger at and envy of the subordinate is not acted on to any significant degree. It is recognized and processed at a mental level and sublimated into generativity. In others, however, it can result in cruel and sadistic verbal attacks or actions intended to impede the development and progression of the protégé.

Attitudes toward money at midlife are closely related to work. For almost all individuals except the very wealthy, the issue is the same—not enough money to meet the extraordinary demands upon the midlife individual to meet daily expenses, to provide children with the opportunity for higher education and/or the transition to independent status, to care for aging parents; and last (unfortunately) but not least, to enjoy oneself in the present and provide for a secure old age.

As with all these developmental tasks, money issues may be a central therapeutic preoccupation, or defensively ignored. In either circumstance, the developmentally oriented therapist, recognizing its importance, will help the middle-aged patient to deal with the powerful thoughts and feelings swirling around finances and to develop realistic plans regarding money management.

PLAY AT MIDLIFE: NEW MEANINGS, ABILITIES, AND PURPOSES

Play is a lifelong human activity, reflecting over the life cycle physical abilities and limitations and mental capabilities and preoccupations. Thus, the unique features of midlife play are, not surprisingly, a reflection of the aging process in the body and the central preoccupation with time limitation and personal death. The form of play does not change much beyond latency and adolescence. The most popular games which adults and children alike prefer, such as baseball, football, golf and tennis, and chess, cards, and board games, are learned before adulthood begins.

By midlife the normal aging processes force the abandonment of most contact sports and the modification of others (walking more and running less, playing doubles rather than singles tennis). Those individuals who cannot accept the aging process in their body often present themselves in therapy with either pathological responses to physical injuries or an exaggerated preoccupation with physical activity—or the reverse, the absence of regular exercise.

In addition to the alterations in play precipitated by the aging body, the psychological *meaning* of sport and exercise also changes. Instead of being used as a joyous expression of physical and mental competence, as it was in childhood and young adulthood, physical forms of play are increasingly associated with maintenance of physical integrity and the enhancement of the aging body. "Use it or lose it" is the slang reflection of this thinking.

Furthermore, both physical and mental forms of play are increasingly used in the service of dealing with the developmental task of accepting time limitation and personal death. Consider golf and gin rummy as examples. Golf is a game full of beginnings and endings; in other words, opportunities to conquer time and imperfection by beginning over and over. There is always another shot, another hole, another match; unlike one's life which has one beginning, and more to the midlife point, an approaching end. Gin rummy and other mental games, which eliminate the necessity to employ the increasingly imperfect body at all, are also built on the same concept of rhythmic beginnings and endings.

An avid golfer patient who was analyzing his admittedly exaggerated response to his game illustrates some of these points. "I got so upset on the course yesterday, I considered quitting for good. Then I thought to myself this is ridiculous; this isn't life or death, it's just a game. I won't even remember what I shot a month from now. I don't want to stop; I love the game. All I have to do is accept a higher handicap as I get older. On second thought, no I don't; when I'm eighty, I want to shoot my age."

MIDLIFE TRANSITION AND CRISIS

Although the terms *midlife transition* and *midlife crisis* have become part of the pop culture, they are definable conditions which have considerable relevance for the clinician. One term, the midlife transition, is a normative, universal developmental phenomenon most often associated with the work of Levinson *et al.* in their book *The Seasons of a Man's Life* (1978). The other, midlife crisis, a term first used by Elliot Jacques (1965) in his article "Death and the Midlife Crisis," refers to a pathological state experienced by only a few individuals.

Transition

The stimuli for both the midlife crisis and transition are the same; namely, the physical, psychological, and environmental changes and pressures just described in the preceding section on developmental tasks; but the responses are very different.

Levinson and his colleagues defined the midlife transition as a reappraisal of all aspects of life precipitated by the growing recognition of time limitation and personal death. It is characterized by thought and feeling, not action. For 80% of the men whom Levinson studied, the examination of relationships, achievements and failures, and future plans was searing in intensity, preoccupying, and painful. For most of the others, this midlife inventory was less conscious and much less painful. The common denominator was the need to assess all aspects of life and make decisions about them—while there was still time to change. For most individuals at midlife (excluding those who experience a midlife crisis), the reappraisal results in decisions to keep most life structures, such as marriages and careers, which have been painstakingly built over time. When changes are made, they are considered and reasonable, even when they include major alterations, such as divorce or job change.

Once again, the developmentally aware clinician recognizes that *every* patient in this age group is engaged in a midlife transition whether the patient is talking about the reappraisal or not.

Nemiroff and I described a true midlife crisis as

a major and revolutionary turning point in one's life, involving changes in
commitments to career and/or spouse and accompanied by significant and
ongoing emotional turmoil for both the individual and others. In addition, the
individual usually feels "unwell" in a context of uncertainty, anxiety, agitation,
or depression. It is an upheaval of major proportions. One woman, on living
through a midlife crisis, precipitated in part by divorce from her husband
described it as "the death of our family as we have known it." (Colarusso &
Nemiroff, 1981, p. 121)

Crisis

After a period of internal agitation, the midlife crisis usually begins
with a flood of action which produces profound change; for example,
leaving spouse and children, becoming involved with a new sexual partner and quitting a job, all within days of each other. Although there may
have been warning signs, those who are left behind are often shocked by
the suddenness and abruptness of the change.

Efforts by family members, or therapists, to get the individual to stop
and consider usually fall on deaf ears. The overwhelming need is to
avoid friends and family who would counsel restraint, and to ignore
therapists who recommend the examination of motivations and feelings
before making such major changes. Usually, during the midst of the
crisis, the therapist is left with the painful job of helping those who have
been left to deal with their shock and grief.

The following description of his crisis was obtained from a man
approximately 18 months after it occurred. Dr. C. was a prominent,
45-year-old physician who had been married 22 years and was the father
of three adolescent children. One Saturday he left home for a weekly
round of golf with friends and did not return. Although he had been
somewhat bored with his wife for some time, he had not made plans to
leave her. As he recalled his thinking, he was standing on the tee on the
tenth hole, after making a par on the ninth, when the thought popped
into his mind that he was not going back—ever again. After showering
and having a drink with his friends he drove 100 miles away and checked
into a motel. He spent the next day in thought "about my life, its meaning and purpose. I suddenly knew it wasn't right for me and I had to
change it." On Monday morning he drove to his home, left his wife a
note in the mailbox telling her, without any explanation, that he was
leaving, and drove to his office. Refusing to accept his wife's frantic calls,
he saw his patients, went to the bank and cashed in a $100,000 certificate
of deposit from his pension plan, and got on a plane for San Diego. Upon
arriving, he left a message on the answering machine of one of his

partners asking him to take over his practice. For the next two months he did nothing but run on the beach and think. Eventually, he wrote his wife a letter telling her where he was and of his decision to remain away.

When he asked to see me 16 months later, he was working in an emergency room and had begun a relationship with a 43-year-old divorcée with two teenaged sons, "not so very different from the family I left," he said.

Our therapeutic efforts to reconstruct his thinking during the acute phase of the crisis were unsuccessful, not because he did not want to, but because he remembered little of his thoughts at the time. He just knew he *had* to change, *now*.

Although we were able to explore the probable dynamics behind the crisis—the recent death of his father, occasional impotence and dissatisfaction with his wife—Dr. C. had no desire to return to his former life. He refused to meet with his wife and eventually agreed to a divorce settlement which gave her almost all of their assets. He did see his children sporadically but did not initiate contacts with them. All of his energies were directed toward "doing what I want to do, meeting new people, and finding myself."

The therapy, which was extremely frustrating for the therapist because of the patient's lack of interest in introspection and his refusal to even consider rebuilding relationships with his wife, children, and extended family, seemed to meet the patient's need to understand himself and build a new life. He eventually married the divorcée and supported his new family by continuing to work in emergency rooms, making far less money than he did in his former practice. He even took up golf again.

Another detailed description of a midlife crisis may be found in *Adult Development* (Colarusso & Nemiroff, 1981) on pages 125–128.

THERAPY WITH MIDLIFE ADULTS

Should the therapist treat the midlife patient differently from any other? The answer is both no and yes. No, in terms of employing standard therapeutic approaches and methods; yes, in terms of conceptualization. Recently Roger Gould (1990) suggested a model of therapy which shifts the therapeutic focus toward the entities of the life cycle without sacrificing the insights which are gained from exploring the patient's past. Gould's model is based on four overlapping but distinct frames of therapeutic reference and activity.

1. The *existential* frame of reference is profoundly influenced by the

issue of time and limitation. Within it therapist and patient consider the meaning and purpose of life and contemplate decisions which will affect the future in some unknown way.

2. Conflicts dealing with immediate life situations are dealt with within the *contextual/developmental* frame of reference. These conflicts are driven by the powerful developmental themes of midlife and require new behavior(s) to bring about successful adaptation.

3. The *developmental/psychodynamic* frame of reference considers the relationship between past influences, conflicts, and inhibitions and the present.

4. Recovery of function and successful adaptation to an adult situation within a *volitional conflict* framework occurs when past memories and present conceptions compete to determine what action will occur, resulting in a new and lasting transformation.

CHAPTER 12

Late and Late Late Adulthood (Age 60 and beyond)

INTRODUCTION

The elderly are the fastest growing segment of the population yet, until recently, the study of their development and methods of treatment specifically suited to them, was neglected. In this chapter, I plan to summarize the most current thinking in the field and point the way to future theoretical and clinical elaboration. The presentation will be divided into four subsections: the developmental tasks of late adulthood, the literature on psychotherapy and psychoanalysis in the second half of life, the nature of psychopathology in late adulthood, and treatment considerations. Material in this chapter is elaborated on in the new edition of the *Course of Life*, edited by Stanley Greenspan and George Pollock. That chapter is entitled "Development and Treatment in Late Adulthood."

THE DEVELOPMENTAL TASKS OF LATE ADULTHOOD

Maintaining the Body Image and Physical Integrity

For many individuals, the passage from youth to old age is mirrored by a shift from the pursuit of wealth to the maintenance of health. Increasingly, the aging body becomes a central intrapsychic concern, replacing the former midlife preoccupations with career and relationships. This is so because of normal diminution in function, altered physical appearance, and the increased incidence of physical illness. Despite these occurrences, the body in late adulthood can still be a source of considerable pleasure and convey a feeling of competence. If attention is paid to regular exercise, healthy diet, and adequate rest, the elderly body can continue to perform many of the physical and mental functions of which it was capable in midlife. The normal state in late adulthood is physical and mental health, not illness and debilitation.

The aging process in late adulthood precipitates significant intrapsychic change, particularly in the body image; that emotionally charged, mental representation of the physical body which is constantly altered throughout the life cycle by actual physical change and evolving demands and expectations. For the most part, the body image closely resembles actual physical appearance; is a source of narcissistic gratification, or injury, depending upon how well it is maintained and functions; and is experienced as an integral part of the psychological sense of self—the basic intrapsychic awareness of "I am."

However, in late adulthood, a *normative dissonance* develops between the body image and the sense of self. As one 70-year-old expressed it upon looking in the mirror, "Who is that impostor staring back at me?" This dissonance is not a reflection of a body image disturbance since the intrapsychic experience of the body closely resembles its actual appearance and functional ability. Rather, it is evidence of a discrepancy between the intrapsychic sense of the body and the sentient self, the latter being experienced as younger and more vigorous, imprisoned, in a sense, in a shell of a body which is no longer compatible with the mind, or able to carry out its commands.

The healthy older person faces the developmental task of recognizing that sooner or later his or her body will become impaired in one or more ways. Then, in the face of either serious physical or mental incapacitation, the elderly individual, and his or her therapist, will face the daunting task of maintaining mental and physical functioning at the highest level possible while mourning for lost functions and altering the body image and sense of self in order to continue living as full and active a life as is possible.

Preparing for Death

Sigmund Freud (1915) described the unmistakable human tendency to eliminate the awareness of death. There is nothing instinctual in us, he noted, which responds to a belief in death; unconsciously we are convinced of our own immortality. Childhood and adolescence are characterized by a tendency to deny the inevitability of death. This denial is bolstered by the anabolic thrust of early development, the immaturity of the psychic apparatus, and the limited understanding of the concept of time (Colarusso, 1987).

In late adolescence, the loosening of ties to the parents combines with experience in living and cognitive maturity to begin to crack the wall of denial, producing in the process a sense of self which includes a more defined past, present, and future (Seton, 1974). But the dawning realization is quickly defended against by youthful idealism and optimism in an attempt, says Jacques (1965), to deny the "two fundamental features of human life—the inevitability of eventual death, and the existence of hate and destructive impulses inside each person" (p. 505).

By middle adulthood, the acceptance of the finiteness of time and the inevitability of personal death has become a central developmental task, forced upon the self by physical aging; the death of parents, friends, and contemporaries; the maturation of children into adulthood; the recognition that not all of life's goals will be realized; and the realization that eventual replacement by younger individuals is inevitable.

By late adulthood *preparation* for death replaces the acceptance of the idea of personal death as the central developmental task. Despite the belief of some that an immutable portion of the self survives, many individuals approach death with considerable protest, manifesting rage at their deity, or themselves, because they have not been made an exception or conquered death on their own (Gottschalk, 1990). For others who have tempered their narcissism to a greater degree, the primary concern is *how* they will die, not if or when. Their fear is that they will die alone or in pain, rather than with a calm dignity in the presence of loved ones.

Accepting the Death of Spouses and Friends

Throughout the life cycle an individual's sense of continuity and sustainment is based on internal representations of self and others. The maintenance of this sense of continuity is both dynamic and developmentally influenced. As Parens (1970) expressed it, "changes in internal representations by the action of assimilative processes effect changes in psychic structure not only in childhood and adolescence, but even in adulthood" (p. 237).

In a long-term marriage, a portion of the self-caregiving is relinquished to the partner. Upon the death of the spouse, two major events occur. First, the identifications which were based on the relationship with the spouse are loosened because they are not continually reinforced by the partner's presence. Second, ongoing identifications are disrupted by the mourning process (Chodorkoff, 1990). Healthy individuals eventually reconstruct a new internal balance of the loved one and new or enhanced relationships with children or friends.

In late adulthood, there is a major intrapsychic difference between being alone and being lonely (Fiske, 1980). The timing of the death of the spouse has a great deal to do with the reaction. If it occurs in old age after a long life and marriage, loneliness may be less intense.

> As family and friends die, move, or become incapacitated, there may be a diminished access to forms of social support that were taken for granted earlier in life. At the same time, with the increased use of reminiscence, first in middle age as a means to solve problems and later in life to provide comfort and preserve a sense of meaning and a continuity of experience, being alone is less disturbing and even desirable, since it allows time for reflection. Despite being foreshortened, the present becomes meaningful through its connection to the past. This connection provides a sense of personal integration. Family and friends may move away or die, memories do not. (Cohler & Galatzer-Levy, 1990)

In the absence of family and upon the death of a spouse, *friendships* may assume a level of importance last seen in adolescence and young adulthood. Similar to the loneliness of young adulthood the loneliness of old age is the result of the absence of committed relationships. A critical difference, however, is based on the fact that young adults have a long future and flexibility spurring them on to form new ties, while the elderly are often impeded by age, illness, and social pressure. Thus, friendships may become the most sustaining relationships available at the end of life, a source of solace and companionship, a receptive ear for the verbalization of the life review, and a hand to hold as death approaches.

Conducting the Life Review

The aging process in the body, the awareness of the finiteness of personal time, and the death of contemporaries are among the influences which stimulate individuals in late life to conduct an intense examination of their lives. Butler (1963) considered the life review to be a prominent developmental process in late adulthood. He and Lewis (1977) defined it as "a universal process brought about by the realization of approaching dissolution and death. It marks the lives of all older persons in some manner as their myths of invulnerability or immortality give way and death begins to be viewed as an immanent personal reality" (p. 165).

A major mental mechanism used in conducting the life review, which is both a conscious and unconscious process, is *reminiscence*. According to Pollock (1981) recollections of the past help the individual to maintain a sense of continuity between past and present, to bridge time, and to enhance a sense of individual personality.

The result of this critical assessment of one's life may be either a sense of integrity or despair (Erikson, 1963). Integrity stems from a realization of having lived life with meaning, fully, and well. Although a sense of meaning to life is highly personal, for Erikson (1973) it involves balancing the certainty of death "with the only happiness that is lasting; to increase, by whatever is yours to give, the good will and higher order in your sector of the world" (p. 124). However, if the life review reveals a series of missed opportunities, bungled relationships, or personal misfortune, the result is a sense of bitter despair and a preoccupation with what might have been. Then death is to be feared, for it symbolizes a life of personal emptiness.

Maintaining Sexual Interests and Activities

Martin (1977) found a steady decrease in the frequency of orgasm, from either coitus or masturbation, with age. Men in their early 30s experienced a peak of 600 sexual events per 5-year period, but by the late 70s, the incidence had dropped to 100 per 5-year period. Harman (1979) described a similar decrease in sexual activity in women. The most important factors in determining the level of sexual activity with age were the health and survival of the spouse; the health of the subject himself or herself; and the level of past sexual activity.

Although some degree of declining sexual interest and function is inevitable with age, social and cultural factors appear to be more responsible for the sexual changes observed than the psychological changes of aging *per se*. Although satisfying sexual activity is possible for the reasonably healthy elderly, many do not actualize this potential. "The widely held view that the elderly are essentially asexual, although it is biologically unsound, is at this time more or less a self-fulfilling prophecy" (Colarusso & Nemiroff, 1961, p. 116).

The major impediments to the continuation of sexual activity in old age are the availability of sexual partners and the attitudes of family members. When partners are available, sexual activity, including intercourse, can continue indefinitely. In the absence of partners, healthy older individuals substitute intercourse with active fantasy lives and masturbation.

The death of a spouse may sometimes have a liberating effect on sexuality. Myers (1991) recently described the reawakening of sexual desire due to alterations in the superego in a 73-year-old man following the death of his wife. According to adult developmental thinking, the ego and superego continue to evolve throughout the life cycle, in adulthood this is due to the waning of the drives and the influence of long-standing object ties, particularly the effect of many years of sexual activity and intimacy with a loved spouse. The death of a spouse is similar to the de-cathexis of the infantile objects during adolescence. Based on loss, real and intrapsychic, both diminish the power of introjects which form the core of the superego. When the inevitability of death is accepted in late adulthood—that intrapsychic process may be stimulated by the death of a spouse—the ego and superego may become more tolerant of sexual thoughts and actions. This may produce a pleasurable increase in sexual activity, or the possibility of reactivated neurotic conflict as wishes or experiences long repressed, or actions formerly inhibited, become conscious and press for expression before death ends the possibility of sexual gratification.

DEVELOPING THE CAPACITY FOR NEW FORMS OF THOUGHT

The Emergence of Wisdom

Labouvie-Vief (1982a,b) suggested that in middle and late adulthood some adults progress beyond formal operations and dialectical thinking (described in Chapter Ten) to the stage of autonomous thought. They can recognize that the thinker participates in creating the truth by understanding the influence of social and personal motivations, thus distinguishing personal and universal reality. Labouvie-Vief described how older adults use a qualitatively different mode of thinking, one which, for instance, considers factors other than the information given to solve a particular problem.

The intellectual behavior of older adults has been described by Edelstein and Noam (1982) as a reunion of logic and affect. This is a prerequisite for the emergence of *wisdom*, that phase-specific mid- and -late-life capacity to understand the long-term consequence of action and to mediate between the demands of logic and emotion.

For some individuals who remain physically and emotionally intact, late and late-late adulthood are the phases of life in which the most sophisticated and complex forms of human thought emerge. Allen Chinen (1984) suggested that this late-life potential is expressed in the ability to experience different modes of logic. Whereas the thinking of midlife is relative and continual, the preoccupation of old age is with universal aspects of truth, including a sense of the infinite and an ability to appreciate the completeness and necessity of individual lives.

RELATIONSHIP TO CHILDREN AND GRANDCHILDREN

The role of parents as facilitators and stimulators of their children's development, continues into late adulthood. Interest in the "child's" family and in their successes in the world continues the pattern of support and love which facilitated the developmental process from birth onward. When the parent has been financially successful, material support of the offspring's family is a prelude to the distribution of accumulated wealth at the time of death.

Grandchildren and great grandchildren are a unique source of pleasure. As the ultimate gift from one's child or grandchild, they offer a new form of immortality by carrying one's genetic material into the future, and through identification, provide an intense psychological focus on the beginning of life as the end of life approaches. The intense, unambivalent love that many grandparents feel toward their grandchildren is based on these factors.

This pattern of the independent parents' facilitating the development of their children and grandchildren may continue throughout this phase into late-late adulthood or it may end sooner, interrupted by change in economic circumstance, illness, or disability. At some point, the elderly parent, no longer able to care for himself or herself, reluctantly accepts the reversal of generations and allows his or her children to become the caretakers and facilitators. The transition, often difficult for the parent and the child, is a frequent theme in clinical work with middle-aged children and their elderly parents. For example, one middle-aged man became caretaker of his somewhat estranged parents when his mother required nursing home care and his father became senile. Resentment over their treatment of him as a child produced great internal conflict as he struggled against the urge to "pay them back." Their decline stimulated the awareness of many previously unavailable memories from childhood which facilitated the therapeutic work.

When parents approach death, feelings between the generations may be stretched to the breaking point and require therapeutic intervention. The reader interested in this subject is referred to the poignant chapter by an expert clinician, Stanley Cath, entitled "When a Wife Dies" (S.H. Cath & C. Cath, 1985, pp. 241–262).

WORK AND RETIREMENT

For some individuals in late adulthood, there is little choice between work and retirement, economic survival requires the former.

Others have an option, albeit a difficult one. But every individual, regardless of circumstance, must accept and integrate the recognition that the end of formal work is approaching, whether due to choice, infirmity, or death.

It may be difficult for the young adult therapist to realize what a consuming psychological preoccupation this is for many individuals approaching or in late adulthood; but an empathetic appreciation will greatly enhance the probabilities of making an accurate diagnosis and conducting successful treatment. Pearl King (1980) suggested that "the threat of redundancy, or displacement in work roles by younger people, and awareness of the possible failure of the effectiveness of their professional skills, linked with the fear that they would not be able to cope with retirement" (p. 154) are among the greatest internal pressures which bring older individuals to treatment.

Transference and countertransference feelings surrounding the patient's work are often difficult and complex. For example, as caring individuals we expect that hard work will be rewarded, that those patients who have spent their adult years in productive work and caring for others will be rewarded by a happy, secure retirement commonly referred to as the "golden years." Yet such is not always the case. Adaptive behaviors in midlife may become maladaptive in late adulthood, and vice versa. For an excellent discussion of these matters, the reader is referred to "The Ant and the Grasshopper in Later Life: Aging in Relation to Work and Gratification" by Ralph Kahana (1985, pp. 263–291). The developmental task becomes the maintenance of a sense of self-worth, relevance, and importance in the absence of traditional work for pay.

Attitudes toward oneself as a mentor and younger workers as mentees occupy a central place in this mid- and late-life transition. The successful mentors gradually recognize that they will eventually be replaced, possibly by a mentee of their own. Hostile wishes toward potential usurpers conflict with wishes to be generative. Developmental progression occurs when the aggression is sublimated into a facilitating teaching role. But the conflict extends not only to the younger individual, but to his or her work as well.

> The capacity to facilitate what is new and valuable independent of its creator must be developed. In the maturing individual, particularly the mentor, this process does not occur easily because of the wish to devalue that which was not created by the self, particularly when time or other limitations reduce the capacity of the self to create. (Nemiroff & Colarusso, 1985, pp. 98–99)

THE LITERATURE ON PSYCHOTHERAPY AND PSYCHOANALYSIS WITH OLDER PATIENTS

Pessimism about the dynamic treatment of older patients began with Sigmund Freud and continues in an unbroken line to the present, despite a growing body of contradictory literature. "Near of above the fifties," said Freud, "the elasticity of the mental process, on which the treatment depends, is as a rule lacking—old people are no longer educable" (1905/1924, p. 264). In addition Freud was concerned that the patient's long past would present the therapist with a "mass" of material too large to analyze. Finally, he was concerned that the patient might die in the near future, choosing cost effectiveness over quality of life. The influence of these ideas has persisted over the decades, in part, because they helped potential therapists of the elderly avoid their concerns about time limitation and personal death.

Kahana (1976) described Freud's dilemma in the following terms:

> Freud was unusually concerned with his own mortality and had an utter and life-long dislike of aging, especially if it entailed any decline in his creativity. In retrospect, these attitudes contrast ironically with his eventual longevity, his remarkable scientific and literary achievements in later life, and his courage in facing prolonged illness and death. (p. 39)

Although Freud revised or discarded many of his ideas, he never changed his opinion about analyzing older patients.

The power of Freud's influence is partly responsible for the relative neglect of the more optimistic findings of Abraham (1949) and Jellifee (1925). Both described great success with older patients, using standard analytic techniques of their day. Jellifee summed up his impressions with the statement "chronological, physiological, and psychological age do not go hand in hand" (p. 9).

Much of the literature of the 1940s and 1950s reflected Freud's viewpoint and emphasized nonanalytic interventions (Alexander & French, 1946; Fenichel, 1945; Hollander, 1952; Wayne, 1953). From the 1960s onward, the literature began to reflect a more optimistic viewpoint (Jacques, 1965; Kahana, 1978; King, 1980; Sandler, 1978). Particularly noteworthy are the contributions of the Boston Society for Gerontological Psychiatry and George Pollock's (1981) description of his work with older patients.

Despite this growing body of literature, many therapists still avoid the elderly. Butler and Lewis (1977) feel this is due to the wish to avoid thinking about old age and personal death and the fear that the patient may die during or soon after the therapy ends. Furthermore, these patients may be organically impaired and therefore untreatable or may stir up conflicts about the therapist's own parents.

ISSUES IN THE TREATMENT OF THE ELDERLY

The implications of the developmental approach for the treatment of the elderly were described with great clarity in the report of the Conference on Psychoanalytic Education and Research (1974) which was sponsored by the American Psychoanalytic Association.

> The implications of the developmental orientation for clinical work stem from the view of individual human development as a continuous and life-long process. One important part of this longitudinal view is the conceptualization of mental illness not in the medical model of disease entities affecting a fully developed organ system, but in the model of functional disturbances which not only impair the current functioning of the individual but impede the development of still-evolving psychic structure and function in one or more of its lines or aspects. By placing mental illness within the broader context of the ongoing process of development we emphasize that the aim of treatment is to enable development to proceed in all of its dimensions. (p. 14)

This statement suggests that the elderly are not removed from the development mainstream but that they, like younger patients, are engaged in developmental conflict, aspects of which are unique to late and late late adulthood, and which can either facilitate developmental progression or produce symptoms. The key to successful treatment lies in the ability of the clinician to focus on *both* the current phase-specific adult developmental issues and the effect of earlier experiences and conflicts, eventually leading to a redefinition and synthesis of the relationship between earlier experience (from childhood and adulthood) and late adult symptomatology and the reengagement of phase-appropriate developmental tasks.

Building on these concepts, Griffin and Grunes (1990) suggested that the reconstruction of self-continuity is the fundamental goal of therapy with the elderly.

> Rather than using therapy as a source of insights about the self, or using the therapeutic relationship as a context to explore new parameters of interpersonal relationships, our experience suggests that the aged use therapy to reconstitute, as much as possible, core bases of selfsameness that have been undermined in later life. (p. 278)

The therapeutic goal of reconstruction is reflected in the patient's successful adaptation to changing realities while reconstituting essential themes from the past. In order for this to occur, the therapist must recognize that memories are vehicles for reviving the viability of the "old" self in the present and the importance of transference as a vehicle for reconstructing a sense of self-continuity.

> If the therapist responds appropriately to the patient's memories (i.e., instead of interpreting them as defensive against the present, the therapist listens with interest and enjoyment), the patient can begin to re-experience the past in the presence of a benign person whose involvement in the memories can revivify them. It is as if the patient can say: Here I can experience myself as I once was, and because I can experience myself in this manner, I must still be the same person. (Griffin & Grunes, 1990, p. 279)

In regard to the use of transference, as the therapist begins to participate in eliciting memories, the patient begins to view him or her as a repository of the younger self. Griffin and Grunes (1990) suggested that therapists not interpret this transference as defensive against the present but use it to forge a new, adaptive integration of past and present.

TRANSFERENCE AND COUNTERTRANSFERENCE

As demonstrated by this example by Griffin and Grunes (1990), transference phenomena in the second half of life are complex and in some aspects qualitatively different from those presented by children and younger adults. This is so because in middle and late adulthood transference phenomena, in addition to being recapitulations of infantile experience, are also expressions of experiences and conflicts from all developmental stages beyond childhood (Shane, 1977).

> Consideration of the impact of psychological development across the life cycle or the experience of remembering the past shows that it is impossible to consider an objective past apart from developmentally determined views of this past which emerge successively during childhood, adolescence, young adulthood, and middle and old age. The fantasies which emerge during the oedipal phase are but prototypes of such developmentally determined fantasies which are associated with each of the phases of development across the life cycle. Review of findings from empirical research on the memorial process at middle age, and of the reminiscence process of life review in old age, suggests that there are fantasies distinctive to phases of development. (Cohler, 1980, pp. 174–175)

Such a conceptualization complicates the therapist's task of understanding and interpreting the transference by suggesting that it is not enough to help the patient recognize the relationship between the infantile past and his or her late adult symptomatology; the contributions of the intervening developmental stages to the symptom complex must also be delineated and analyzed. Furthermore, as described by both Griffin and Grunes, and Cohler, transferences in late adulthood may be expressed through phase-specific developmental themes and concerns, such as the integrity of the self and the life review.

Analysis and management of the transference are also affected when the elderly patient has a limited number of meaningful object ties; for example, if he or she has recently lost a spouse or is separated from children by distance. In these circumstances, the therapeutic relationship may become exceptionally important and undermine the therapeutic effort. Although positive transference may develop very rapidly and be difficult to resolve because the patient does not wish to give up its pleasures, negative transference feelings may be withheld entirely out of fear of abandonment. Some patients will attempt to continue the therapeutic relationship indefinitely, substituting its transference gratifications for the fuller and more lasting pleasures which are available in the real world (Colarusso and Nemiroff, 1991).

Multigenerational Transference

One of the most important studies of transference and countertransference in late adulthood was conducted by Hiatt (1971). In his longitudinal study of patients between the ages of 60 and 84, he delineated several kinds of transference which occur, some resulting from relationships beyond infancy and early childhood. He categorized them as follows:

1. The well-recognized *parental transference,* in which the patient reacts to the therapist as a child to a parent.
2. *Peer or sibling transference,* expressions of experiences from a variety of nonparental relationships.

   > This group looks to the therapist . . . to share experiences of an interpersonal nature involving other members of the family. It may be somewhat startling to the therapist to have his age ignored and be transformed into a most trusted symbol of the patient's spouse, business associate or roommate. (Hiatt, 1971, p. 594)

3. *Son or daughter transference.* In this reversed transference situation, which is extremely common in elderly patients, the therapist is cast in the role of the patient's child, grandchild, or son- or daughter-in-law. The themes expressed in this form of transference are multiple and often are centered around defenses against dependency feelings, activity and dominance versus passivity and submission, and attempts to rework unsatisfying aspects of relationships with children before time runs out.
4. Last, but by no means least, *sexual transferences* in the elderly are frequent, intense, and extremely useful to the therapist who

can accept them and manage his or her countertransference responses.

Detailed case histories illustrating these points have been presented by Cohen (1965), Crusey, (1985), Hildebrand (1985), and Levinson (1985), among others.

Countertransference

In addition to the typical forms of countertransference observed in the treatment of younger patients, some are related to the elderly patient's position in the life cycle. Individuals in late and late-late adulthood are dealing with illness and advanced signs of aging, the loss of spouses and friends, and the constant awareness of time limitation and the nearness of death. These are painful issues which are just beginning to come into focus for middle-aged therapists who would prefer not to confront them with great intensity on a daily basis.

A second source of countertransference response is the therapist's reaction to the elderly patient's sexuality. The presence of a vivid fantasy life, masturbation, and, when a partner is available, intercourse, is disconcerting in and of itself if the therapist has not had much experience in working with individuals in late adulthood, but pale when compared to a strong erotic transference.

Consider some of the comments of Jill Crusey (1985), who was 31 years of age at the time she was treating a 62-year-old man:

> Early in the treatment process, Mr. D.'s sexual feelings emerged. His well-groomed appearance and adolescent-like nervousness in the first half of our sessions prompted a little discomfort on my part. My concern was how to engender respect and develop a therapeutic alliance with a patient who approached each session as a date, particularly a patient who was old enough to be my grandfather.
>
> ... Apparently, it is difficult for a young colleague to imagine that he or she and a parent may have a similar infantile conflict to resolve in spite of a 30-year age difference. Somehow, I wanted Mr. D. to be all grown up, devoid of issues with which I may be grappling also. However, Mr. D. taught me that to ignore the psychodynamics of his conflicts would be to sentence him to a premature death.
>
> Each of these transference situations stimulated the question, How would I feel if it were my father in treatment working through such issues? I found it illuminating to be reminded that he too may have had psychological conflicts. (pp. 165–166)

Another example of countertransference in work with individuals in late adulthood involves sibling issues since the therapist is frequently seen as the patient's child. The transference expresses whatever issues, positive or negative, the patients may have with their child, the counter-transference is based on the therapist's issues with siblings, parents, or children. For example, positive feelings toward the therapist as the ideal son or daughter may complement his or her wish to be the only favored offspring, leading to a mutually gratifying interaction rather than under-standing. In the event of serious illness in the patient's life, the situation may be further complicated by actual involvement with members of the patient's family.

Hiatt (1971) has categorized countertransference reactions to older patients as follows:

1. An omnipotent or unrealistic hope. In an attempt to avoid dealing with his or her own feelings about illness and death, the therapist denies realistic infirmities in the patient.
2. The feeding of one's narcissism and gaining personal gratifica-tion. This involves enjoying, rather than analyzing, the elderly patient's need to overestimate, for defensive purposes, the therapist's knowledge and ability to protect and help the patient.
3. An unreasonable anger and desire to avoid work with the older patient. This countertransference reaction occurs in response to manipulative or regressive behavior in the elderly patient, and may not be based on past or current interactions with one's own parents.
4. The feeling of pity and sorrow for a person at the end of life. This conscious feeling may cover death wishes toward parents (from infantile or adult experience) and lead to an avoidance of the phase-specific need on the part of the elderly patients to discuss their attitudes about death.

SPECIAL TECHNIQUES FOR WORKING WITH THE ELDERLY

George Pollock: The Therapeutic Value of Reminiscence

Recognizing that loss is a universal experience which has consider-able effect on psychic processes, Pollock (1979) elaborated a theory of mourning and described the usefulness of reminiscence in work with patients. Mourning, he suggested, is a transformational process which allows us to accept painful aspects of reality and which produces recog-nizable intrapsychic and real changes. Focusing on the mourning process in therapy helps the patient recognize and accept the loss of parts of the self that once were. As lost objects, hopes and aspirations are analyzed and accepted, and new sublimations, interests, and relationships can be considered and pursued.

Reminiscence is particularly valuable in the elderly because it helps them maintain a sense of self and a connectedness between past and present in the face of a growing awareness of diminished ego intactness and competency. Depending on the patient, the focus on the past may be a form of mourning or a working through of past conflicts. In either event, "the insight of the psychoanalytic observer allows for understanding the meaning of what is otherwise considered 'the ramblings of old men and women'" (Pollock, 1981, p. 280).

The Life Review in Therapy

Conducting a life review was described earlier in the chapter as an important, phase-specific, developmental task of late adulthood. This effort is often an integral part of the therapeutic process with the elderly, particularly if the therapist chooses to utilize some of the techniques described by Butler and Lewis (1977). They suggested asking the patient to organize an outline for an autobiography. This effort provides the therapist with new information and allows him or her to look for experiences which are emphasized or avoided. In addition, Butler and Lewis encouraged visits to important people and places from the past. Class reunions would be an example. Such experiences sharpen the distinction between past and present by facilitating mourning and providing an opportunity to reconnect with those real aspects of the past which still exist. Genealogy and the preservation of personal, ethic, and cultural identity through the examination of scrapbooks and albums, as well as more formal investigations, are all therapeutically useful when studied together by the therapist and the patient.

Techniques for Treating the Debilitated Elderly

Goldfarb (1955, 1967) and Goldfarb and Sheps (1954) described techniques for treating those individuals, usually residents of nursing homes, who have suffered profound physical and/or psychological impairment. They noted that these individuals often reacted to their increasing helplessness by attempting to dominate and control others, including the therapist, or by developing a childlike dependent transference. Using these insights, Goldfarb and Sheps suggested the following therapeutic strategies:

> By utilizing the role that the security seeking aged sick force on him, guilt, fear, rage and depression can be ameliorated or their social manifestations

altered. The patient's sense of helplessness is then decreased. Some successes in performance which follow tend to further increase the patient's sense of worth and strength. Therapy consists of brief (five to fifteen minutes) sessions which are as widely spaced as the status and progress of the patient permits. Each of the interviews is "structured" so that the patient leaves with a sense of triumph, or victory derived from having won an ally or from having dominated the therapist. The therapist attempts to have the patient leave not with the feeling of guilt but of conquest (triumph). (p. 183)

Influencing the attitudes of the staff who care for the debilitated elderly is an essential aspect of the therapist's task. How to accomplish this difficult and complicated task was vividly described by Cohen (1985) in his psychotherapeutic treatment of an 80-year-old patient whom he followed for several years, both before and after a major stroke which left her severely demented.

Mrs. C. had not only lost touch with her personal history, but she had also lost her ability to convey her own history to others. In this regard, we all have a compound history, a two-faceted history—a history of ourselves as we know it and a history of ourselves as others know it. Not to be known by others, to be in effect without a history by being unable to convey one's past, puts a person at a severe disadvantage in eliciting the understanding and empathy of others; a competitive edge has been lost. Here, the therapist can be enormously helpful in conveying the individual's personal and dynamic history, his or her clinical biography. I then attempted to restore some of this competitive edge, this most interesting human phenomena—Mrs. C.'s history, her biography. Scrapbooks, photos, news clippings, and other personal items of memorabilia were gathered in the process of trying to portray a sense of the patient's past to the staff dynamically. The impact was pronounced. When I returned the next week, there was considerably more verbal and non-verbal engagement between the staff and Mrs. C. And, as more time passed, it became apparent that in addition to the staff's feeling more in touch with the patient because of their knowledge of her personal history, fragments of disjointed thoughts she would express were somewhat better understood due to the enlarged frame of reference in which they were heard.

The problem of imparting Mrs. C.'s history was a much more complicated idea than what has been described. This was because of the dual problem of there being more than one shift of personnel during the course of each day and substantial staff turnover (particularly nursing assistants at the nursing homes) during the course of the year. How, then, can one practically convey the patient's history in the dynamic manner described for each shift and for ongoing new staff? Certainly, it is difficult to achieve this effect with a typical chart history; the length involved might preclude many from reading it. It was felt then that one could take advantage of the new technology of audio and videocassettes and record the history on one or the other of these media. For some institutions there would be the resources to develop a program of audiovisual histories. In other settings, the costs might be prohibitive, but audiocassette histories could still be feasible. Staff at all shifts might be much more likely to obtain these histories due to ease of access-listening to or watching a cassette presentation as opposed to pondering over a chart. Family members could also assume an important role here and probably derive much satisfaction by contributing to the information and presentation on the cassettes. Especially if a given family member is a good storyteller, they should be involved in giving the patient's biography. The experience could be rewarding all the way around. And, in this case example, it might be appreciated that in patients with severe dementia the role of biography can be as important as that of biology in the overall approach to treatment. (pp. 202–203)

References

Abraham, K. 1949. The applicability of psycho-analytic treatment to patients at an advanced age. In *Selected Papers of Psychoanalysis*. London: Hogarth Press.

Abrams, S. 1978. The teaching and learning of psychoanalytic developmental psychology. *J. Amer. Psychoanal. Assn.* 26:387–396.

Alexander, F. G., & French, T. M. 1946. *Psychoanalytic Therapy: Principles and Applications*. London: Ronald Press.

American Psychiatric Association. 1987. *Diagnostic and Statistical Manual of Mental Disorders*. (3rd ed., rev.). Washington, D.C.: American Psychiatric Association.

Anthony, E. J. 1982. Normal adolescent development from a cognitive viewpoint. *J. Amer. Acad. Child Psychiat.* 21:318–327.

Arnstein, R. L. 1980. The student, the family, the university, and transition to adulthood. In *Adolescent Psychiatry* (S.C. Feinstein, ed.). Chicago: University of Chicago Press.

Back, K. W. 1974. Transition to aging and the self image. In *Normal Aging: Vol. II* (E. Palmore, Ed.). Durham: Duke University Press, pp. 207–216.

Bardwick, J. M. 1986. *The Plateauing Trap*. New York: American Management Association.

Basseches, M. 1984. *Dialectic Thinking and Adult Development*. Norwood: Ablex.

Berman, E. M., & Lief, H. I. 1975. Marital therapy from a psychiatric perspective: An overview. *Amer. J. Psychiatry* 132:6–19.

Bettelheim, B. 1976. *The Uses of Enchantment: The Meaning and Importance of Fairy Tales*. London: Thames and Hudson.

Block, J. 1971. *Lives Through Time*. Berkeley: Bancroft Books.

Blos, P. 1962. *On Adolescence: A Psychoanalytic Interpretation*. New York: Free Press.

Blos, P. 1967. The second individuation process of adolescence. *Psychoanal. Study Child* 22:162–186.

Blos, P. 1970. *The Young Adolescent: Clinical Studies*. New York: Free Press.

Blos, P. 1974. The genealogy of the ego ideal. *Psychoanal. Study Child* 29:43–88.

Blos, P. 1979. *The Adolescent Passage*. New York: International Universities Press.

Bornstein, B. 1951. On latency. *Psychoanal. Study Child* 5:279–286.

Bornstein, B. 1953. Fragment of an analysis of an obsessional child: The first six months of analysis. *Psychoanal. Study Child* 8:313–332.

Brunswick, R. M. 1940. The preoedipal phase of libido development. *Psychoanal. Quart.* 9:293–307.

Butler, R. N. 1963. The life review: An interpretation of reminiscence in the aged. *Psychiatry* 26:65–76.

Butler, R. N. & Lewis, M. I. 1977. *Aging and Mental Health: Positive Psychosocial Approaches.* St. Louis: Mosby.

Cath, S. H., & Cath, C. 1985. When a wife dies. In *The Race against Time: Psychotherapy and Psychoanalysis in the Second Half of Life* (R. Nemiroff and C. Colarusso, Eds.). New York: Plenum Press, pp. 241–262.

Cath, S. H., Gurwitt, A. R., & Ross, J. M. (Eds.). 1982. *Father and Child: Developmental and Clinical Perspectives.* Boston: Little, Brown.

Cath, S. H., Gurwitt, A. R., & Gunsberg, L. (Eds.). 1989. *Fathers and Their Families,* Hillsdale, The Analytic Press.

Chinen, A. B. 1984. Modal logic, a new paradigm of development and late life potential. *Human Development* 27:52–56.

Chodorkoff, B. 1990. The catastrophic reaction: Developmental aspects of a severe reaction to loss in later life. In: *New Dimensions in Adult Development* (R. Nemiroff & C. Colarusso, Eds.). New York: Basic Books, pp. 371–385.

Clower, V. L. 1976. Theoretical implications in current views of masturbation in latency girls. *J. Amer. Psychoanal. Assn.* 24:109–126.

Cohen, J. 1985. Psychotherapy with an eighty-year-old patient. In: *The Race against Time: Psychotherapy and Psychoanalysis in the Second Half of Life* (R. Nemiroff & C. Colarusso, Eds.). New York: Plenum Press, pp. 195–210.

Cohler, B. J. 1980. Adult Developmental Psychology and Reconstruction in Psychoanalysis. In *The Course of Life: Psychoanalytic Contributions Toward Understanding Personality Development, Vol. III,* S. J. Greenspan & G. H. Pollock, eds. Washington, D.C.: U.S. Government Printing Office, DHHS Publication No. (ADM) 81-1000, pp. 149–199.

Cohler, J., & Lieberman, M. 1979. Personality change across the second half of life. Findings from a study of Irish, Italian, and Polish-American Men and Women. In: *Ethnicity and Aging* (D. Gelfand & A. Kutznik, eds.). New York: Springer, pp. 227–245.

Cohler, B. L., & Galatzer-Levy, R. M. 1990. Self, meaning, and morale across the second half of life. In: *New Dimensions in Adult Development* (R. Nemiroff & C. Colarusso, Eds.). New York: Basic Books, pp. 214–263.

Colarusso, C. A. 1979. The development of time sense—from birth to object constancy. *Int. J. Psychoanal.* 60:243–252.

Colarusso, C. A. 1987. The development of time sense—from object constancy to adolescence. *J. Amer. Psychoanal. Assn.* 35:119–144.

Colarusso, C. A. 1988. The development of time sense in adolescence. *Psychoanal. Study Child* 43:179–198.

Colarusso, C. A. 1990. The third individuation: The effect of biological parenthood on separation-individuation processes in adulthood. *Psychoanal. Study Child* 45:170–194.

Colarusso, C. A. In press. Traversing Young Adulthood: The Male Journey from Twenty to Forty. *Psychoanalytic Inquiry.*

Colarusso, C. A., & Nemiroff, R. A. 1981. *Adult Development: A New Dimension in Psychodynamic Theory and Practice.* New York: Plenum Press.

Colarusso, C. A., & Nemiroff, R. A. 1982. The father in midlife: Crisis and growth of paternal identity. In *Father and Child* (S. H. Cath, A. Gurwitt, & J. M. Ross, Eds.). Boston: Little, Brown, pp. 315–328.

Colarusso, C. A., & Nemiroff, R. A. 1991. Impact of adult developmental issues on treatment of older adults. In: *New Techniques in the Psychotherapy of Older Patients* (W. Myers, Ed.). Washington, D.C.: American Psychiatric Press, pp. 245–265.

Commons, M. L., & Richards, F. A. 1982. A general model of stage theory. In: *Beyond Formal Operations: Late Adolescent and Adult Cognitive Development* (M. L. Commons, F. A. Richards, & S. Armon, Eds.). New York: Praeger.

Conference on Psychoanalytic Education and Research, Commission IX. 1974. *Child Analysis*. New York: American Psychoanalytic Association.

Cooper, A. M. 1985. Will Neurobiology Influence Psychoanalysis? *American Journal of Psychiatry* 142:1395–1402.

Crusey, J. E. 1985. Short-term psychodynamic psychotherapy with a sixty-two-year-old man. In: *The Race against Time* (R. Nemiroff & C. Colarusso, Eds.). New York: Plenum Press, pp. 147–170.

Dowling, S., & Rothstein, A. (Eds.). 1989. *The Significance of Infant Observational Research for Clinical Work with Children, Adolescents, and Adults*. Madison: International Universities Press.

Edelstein, W., & Noam, G., 1982. Regulatory structures of self and post-formal stages in adulthood. *Human Development* 25:407–422.

Edgcumbe, R., & Burgner, M. 1975. The phallic-narcissistic phase: A differentiation between preoedipal and oedipal aspects of phallic development. *Psychoanal. Study Child* 30:161–180.

Eichorn, D. A., Clausen, J. A., & Haan, H. 1981. *Present and Past in Middle Life*. New York: Academic Press.

Eisdorfer, C., & Raskind, R. 1975. Aging and human behavior. In B. E. Eleftreriois & R. L. Spatts (Eds.), *Hormonal Correlates of Behavior, Vol 1. A Lifespan View*. New York: Plenum Press, pp. 369–387.

Eissler, K. 1975. On possible effects of aging on the practice of psychoanalysis: An essay, *J. Phila. Assoc. Psychoanal.* 11:139–176.

Emde, R. N. 1985. From adolescence to midlife: Remodeling the structure of adult development. *J. Amer. Psychoanal. Assn.* 33:59–112.

Erikson, E. H. 1956. The concept of ego identity. *J. Amer. Psychoanal. Assn.* 4:56–121.

Erikson, E. H. 1963. *Childhood and Society*, 2nd ed. New York: W. W. Norton.

Erikson, E. H. 1973. *Dimensions of a New Identity: Jefferson Lectures*. New York: W. W. Norton.

Fenichel, O. 1945. *The Psychoanalytic Theory of Neurosis*. New York: W. W. Norton.

Fiske, M. 1980. Tasks and crises of the second half of life: The interrelationship of commitment, coping, and adaptation. In: *Handbook of Health and Aging* (J. Burren & R. B. Sloan, Eds.). Englewood Cliffs, Prentice Hall, pp. 337–373.

Ferenczi, S. 1913. Stages in the development of the sense of reality. *Int. Z. Psychoanal.*

Freud, A. 1936, *The Ego and Mechanisms of Defense*. In: *The Writing of Anna Freud* (Vol. 2, rev. ed.). New York: International Universities Press.

Freud, A. 1946. The psychoanalytic study of infant feeding disturbances. *Psychoanal. Study Child* 2:119–132.

Freud, A. 1958. Adolescence. *Psychoanal. Study Child* 13:255–278.

Freud, A. 1965. *Normality and Pathology in Childhood: Assessments of Development*. New York: International Universities Press.

Freud, A. 1981. The concept of developmental lines: Their diagnostic significance. *Psychoanal. Study Child* 36:129–136.

Freud, A., Nagera, H., & Freud, W. E. 1965. Metapsychological assessment of the adult personality. *Psychoanal. Study Child* 20:9–41.

Freud, S. 1905. Three essays on the theory of sexuality. In: *Standard Edition* (J. Strachey, Ed., 1968), 7:125–243. London: Hogarth Press.

Freud, S. 1909. Analysis of a phobia in a five-year-old boy. In: *The Standard Edition* (J. Strachey, Ed., 1958), 10:3–148, London: Hogarth Press.

Freud, S. 1911. Formulations on the two principles of mental functioning. In: *The Standard Edition* (J. Strachey, Ed., 1958), 12:213–218. London: Hogarth Press.

Freud, S. 1912. The dynamics of transference. In: *The Standard Edition* (J. Strachey, Ed.). 7:98–108. London: Hogarth Press.

Freud, S. 1914. On narcissism. In: *The Standard Edition* (J. Strachey, Ed., 1958), 14:67–102. London: Hogarth Press.

Freud, S. 1915. Thoughts for the times on war and death. In: *The Standard Edition* (J. Strachey, Ed., 1958), 14:273–301. London: Hogarth Press.

Freud, S. 1918. From the history of an infantile neurosis. In: *The Standard Edition* (J. Strachey, Ed., 1958), 17:3–122. London: Hogarth Press.

Freud, S. 1921. Group psychology and the analysis of the ego. In: *The Standard Edition* (J. Strachey, Ed., 1958). 18:67–143. London: Hogarth Press.

Freud, S. 1923. Ego and the id. In: *The Standard Edition* (J. Strachey, Ed., 1958), 19:3–66. London: Hogarth Press.

Freud, S. 1924a. On psychotherapy. In *Collected papers* (Vol. 1). London: Hogarth Press. (Originally published, 1905).

Freud, S. 1924b. The dissolution of the Oedipal complex. In: *The Standard Edition* (J. Strachey, Ed., 1968), 19:172–179. London: Hogarth Press.

Freud, S. 1930. Civilization and its discontents. In: *The Standard Edition* (J. Strachey, Ed.), 21:59–246. London: Hogarth Press.

Freud, S. 1940. An outline of psycho-analysis. In: *The Standard Edition* (J. Strachey, Ed., 1968), 23:141–207. London: Hogarth Press.

Galenson, E., & Roiphe, H. 1974. The emergence of genital awareness during the second year of life. In: *Sexual Differences in Behavior* (R. C. Friedman, Ed.). New York: Wiley, pp. 223–231.

Galenson, E., & Roiphe, H. 1976. Some suggested revisions concerning early female development. *J. Amer. Psychoanal. Assn. Supplement, Female Psychology #5*, 24:29–58.

Gesell, A., & Ilg, F. L. 1943. *Infant and Child in the Culture of Today.* New York: Harper.

Glover, E. 1945. Examination of the Klein system of child psychology. *Psychoanal. Study Child* 1:78–93.

Goin, M. K. 1990. Emotional survival and the aging body. In: *New Dimensions In Adult Development* (R. Nemiroff and C. Colarusso, Eds.). New York: Basic Books, pp. 518–531.

Goldfarb, A. L. 1955. One aspect of the psychodynamics of the therapeutic situation with aged patients. *Psychoanalytic Review* 42:180–187.

Goldfarb, A. L. 1967. *Psychiatry in Geriatrics, Medical Clinics of North America.* Philadelphia: W. B. Saunders.

Goldfarb, A. L., & Sheps, J. 1954. Psychotherapy of the aged. *Psychosomatic Medicine* 15:3–12.

Gottschalk, L. A. 1990. Origins and evolution of narcissism through the life cycle. In: *New Dimensions in Adult Development* (R. Nemiroff & C. Colarusso, Eds.). New York: Basic Books.

Gould, R. L. 1978. *Transformations: Growth and Change in Adult Life.* New York: Simon & Schuster.

Gould, R. L. 1990. Clinical lessons from adult developmental therapy. In: *New Dimensions in Adult Development* (R. Nemiroff & C. Colarusso, Eds.). New York: Basic Books, pp. 345–370.

Greenacre, P. 1953. Penis awe and its relation to penis envy. In: *Emotional Growth* (Vol. I). New York: International Universities Press, pp. 31–49.

Greenson, R. R. 1954. The struggle against identification. *J. Amer. Psychoanal. Assn.* 2:200–217.

Greenspan, S. I., & Pollock, G. H. 1981. *The Course of Life: Contributions toward Understanding Personality Development, Infancy and Early Childhood* (Vol. I); *Latency, Adolescence, and Youth* (Vol. II); and *Adulthood and Aging* (Vol. III). Washington, D.C.: Government Printing Office.

Griffin, B. P., & Grunes, J. M. 1990. A developmental approach to psychoanalytic psycho-therapy with the aged. In: *New Dimensions in Adult Development* (R. Nemiroff & C. Colarusso, Eds.). New York: Basic Books, pp. 267–287.

Gurwitt, A. 1982. Aspects of prospective fatherhood. In: *Father and Child* (S. Cath, A. Gurwitt, and J. M. Ross, Eds.), Boston: Little, Brown, pp. 275–300.

Gutmann, D. 1971. Cross-cultural research on human behavior: A comparative study of the life cycle in the middle and later years. In: *Environmental Influences and Genetic Expression* (N. Kretchmer & F. Walcher, Eds.). Washington, D.C.: Government Printing Office, Fogarty International Center Proceedings, No. 2.

Guttman, D. 1977. Parenthood: A comparative key to the life-cycle. In: *Life-Span Developmental Psychology: Normative Life Crises* (N. Datan & L. Ginsberg, Eds.). New York: Academic Press, pp. 167–184.

Guttman, D. 1987, *Reclaimed Powers: Toward a Psychology of Men and Women in Later Life*. New York: Basic Books.

Guttman, D. 1990. Psychological Development and Pathology in Later Life. In *New Dimensions in Adult Development* (R. Nemiroff & C. Colarusso, eds.) New York: Basic Books, pp. 170–185.

Guttman, D., Griffin, B., & Grunes, J., 1982. Developmental contributions to the late-onset affective disorders. In: *Life-Span Development and Behavior* (P. Baltes & O. G. Brim, Jr., Eds.). New York: Academic Press, pp. 244–263.

Harman, S. W. 1979. Male menopause? The hormones flow but sex goes slow. *Medical World News* 20:11–18.

Hartmann, H. 1964. *Essays on Ego Psychology*. Princeton: Princeton University Press.

Heath, R. 1979. *Princeton Retrospective: The Class of 1954*. Princeton: Princeton University Press.

Hertzog, J. M. 1982. Patterns of expectant fatherhood: A study of the fathers of a group of premature infants. In: *Father and Child* (S. Cath, A. Gurwirr, & J. M. Ross, Eds.). Boston: Little, Brown, pp. 301–314.

Hertzog, J. M. 1984. Fathers and young children: Fathering daughters and fathering sons. In: *Frontiers of Infant Psychiatry* (J. D. Call, E. Galenson, & R. L. Tyson, Eds.). New York: Basic Books, pp. 335–342.

Hiatt, H. 1971. Dynamic psychotherapy with the aging patient. *American J. Psychotherapy* 25:591–600.

Hildebrand, H. P. 1985. Object loss and development in the second half of life. In: *The Race against Time* (R. Nemiroff & C. Colarusso, Eds.). New York: Plenum Press, pp. 311–328.

Hollander, M. H. 1952. Individualizing the aged. *Social Casework* 33:99–116.

Horney, K. 1924. On the genesis of the castration complex in women. In: *Feminine Psychology* (H. Kelman, Ed.). New York: W. W. Norton, 1967, pp. 37–53.

Jacobson, E. 1961. Adolescent moods and the remodeling of psychic structure in adolescence. *Psychoanal. Study Child* 16:164–183.

Jacques, E. 1965. Death and the midlife crisis. *Int. J. Psychoanal.* 46:502–514.

Jarvik, L. J., Eisdofer, C., & Blum, J. E. 1973. *Intellectual Functioning in Adults*. New York: Springer.

Jellifee, S. E. 1925. The old age factor in psycho-analytic therapy. *Medical Journal Records* 121:7–12.

Jung, C. G. 1933. *Modern Man in Search of a Soul*. New York: Harcourt, Brace.

Kahana, R. 1978. Psychoanalysis in later life. Discussion. *J. Geriatric Psych.* 11:37–49.

Kahana, R. 1985. The ant and the grasshopper in later life: Aging in relationship to work and gratification. In: *The Race against Time* (R. Nemiroff & C. Colarusso, Eds.). New York: Plenum Press, pp. 263–292.

Kandel, E. R. 1976. *Cellular Bases of Behavior: An Introduction to Behavioral Neurology.* New York: W. H. Freeman.

Kandel, E. 1986. Book Review. In *Psychotherapy and Social Sciences.* Northvale, N.J.: Jason Aronson, p. 36.

Kandel, E. R., & Schwartz, J. H. 1982. Molecular biology of learning: Modulation of transmitter release. *Science,* 218:433–442.

Kanner, L. 1943. Autistic disturbances of affective contact. *Nerv. Child* 2:21–250.

Kaplan, E. B. 1965. Reflections regarding psychomotor activities during the latency period. *Psychoanal. Study Child* 20:220–238.

Katan, A. 1961. Some thoughts about the role of verbalization in childhood. *Psychoanal. Study Child* 16:184–188.

Katz, A. 1968. *No Time for Youth.* San Francisco: Jossey-Bass.

Kernberg, O. F. 1976. *Borderline Conditions and Pathologic Narcissism.* New York: Jason Aronson.

Kestenberg, J. 1968. Outside and inside, male and female. *J. Amer. Psychoanal. Assn.* 16:457–520.

Kestenberg, J. 1976. Regression and reintegration in pregnancy. *J. Amer. Psychoanal. Assn. Supplement, Female Psychology #5,* 24:213–250.

King, P. 1980. The life cycle as indicated by the nature of the transference in the psychoanalysis of the middle-aged and elderly. *Int. J. Psychoanal.* 61:153–160.

Kleeman, J. A. 1966. Genital self-discovery during a boy's second year: A follow-up. *Psychoanal. Study Child* 21:358–392.

Kohut, H. 1971. *The Analysis of the Self: A Systematic Approach to the Psychoanalytic Treatment of Narcissistic Personality Disorders.* New York: International Universities Press.

Kohut, H. 1977. *Restoration of the Self.* New York: International Universities Press.

Kramer, S., & Akhtar, S. 1988. The developmental context of internalized preoedipal object relations: Clinical applications of Mahler's theory of symbiosis and separation–individuation. *Psychoanal. Quart.* 57:547–576.

Labouvie-Vief, G. 1982a. Dynamic development and mature autonomy. *Human Development* 25:161–191.

Labouvie-Vief, G. 1982b. Growth and aging in life-span perspective. *Human Development* 25:65–78.

Levinson, D. J., Darrow, C. N., & Klein, E. B. 1978. *The Seasons of a Man's Life.* New York: Alfred A. Knopf.

Levinson, G. 1985. New beginnings at seventy: A decade of psychotherapy in late adulthood. In: *The Race against Time* (R. Nemiroff & C. Colarusso, Eds.). New York: Plenum Press, pp. 171–194.

Lieberman, M., & Tobin, S. 1983. *The Experience of Old Age: Stress, Coping, and Survival.* New York: Basic Books.

Loewald, H. 1985. Oedipal complex and the development of the self. *Psychoanal. Quart.* 54:435–443.

Loewald, H. W. 1979. The waning of the Oedipal Complex. In: *Papers on Psychoanalysis.* New Haven: Yale University Press, pp. 384–404.

Mahler, M. 1952. On child psychosis and schizophrenia: Autistic and symbiotic infantile psychosis. *Psychoanal. Study Child* 7:286–305.

Mahler, M. 1958. From autism to symbiosis. *Int. J. Psychoanal.* 39:83–92.

Mahler, M. 1963. Thoughts about development and individuation. *Psychoanal. Study Child* 18:307–324.

Mahler, M. 1967. On human symbiosis and the vicissitudes of individuation. *J. Amer. Psychoanal. Assn.* 15:740–763.

Mahler, M., Pine, F., & Bergman, A. 1975. *The Psychological Birth of the Human Infant*. New York: Basic Books.

Martin, C. E. 1977. Sexual activity in the aging male. In: *Handbook of Sexuality* (J. Money & H. Musaph, Eds.). Amsterdam: Elsevier/North-Holland.

Maslow, A. H. 1968. *Toward a Psychology of Being*. New York: Van Nostrand.

Masters, W., & Johnson, V. 1966. *Human Sexual Response*. Boston: Little, Brown.

Moore, B. E., & Fine, B. D. (Eds.). 1990. *Psychoanalytic Terms and Concepts* (The American Psychoanalytic Association). New Haven: Yale University Press.

Myers, W. (Ed.). 1991. *New Techniques in the Psychotherapy of Older Patients*. Washington, D.C.: American Psychiatric Press.

Nagera, H. 1966. Sleep and its disturbances approached developmentally. *Psychoanal. Study Child* 21:393–447.

Nemiroff, R. A., & Colarusso, C. A. 1985. *The Race against Time: Psychotherapy and Psychoanalysis in the Second Half of Life*. New York: Plenum Press.

Nemiroff, R. A., & Colarusso, C. A. (Eds.). 1990. *New Dimensions in Adult Development*. New York: Basic Books.

Neugarten, B., 1979. Time, age and the life cycle. *Amer. J. Psychiatry* 136:887–894.

Neugarten, B. L. 1975. Adult personality: Toward a psychology of the life cycle. In: *The Human Life Cycle* (W. C. Sze, Ed.). New York: Jason Aronson.

Neugarten, B. L., Berkowitz, H., Crotty, W. J., Gruen, W., Gutmann, D. L., Lubin, M. I., Miller, D. L., Peck, R. F., Rosen, J. L., Shukin, A., & Tobin, S. S. 1964. *Personality in Middle and Late Life*. New York: Atherton Press.

Offer, D., & Offer, J. B. 1975. *From Teenage to Young Manhood: A Psychological Study*. New York: Basic Books.

Offer, D., & Sabshin, M. (Eds.). 1984. *Normality and the Life Cycle*. New York: Basic Books.

Oldham, J. M., & Liebert, R. S. 1989. *The Middle Years*. New Haven: Yale University Press.

Panel, 1973a. The experience of separation-individuation in infancy and its reverberations through the course of life: Infancy and childhood. M. Winestine, reporter. *J. Psychoanal. Assn.* 12:135–154.

Panel, 1973b. The experience of separation-individuation through the course of life: Adolescence and maturity. J. Marcus, reporter. *J. Amer. Psychoanal. Assn.* 21:155–167.

Parens, H. 1970. Inner sustainment: Metaphysical considerations. *Psychoanal. Quart.* 39:223–239.

Pearson, G. 1958. *Adolescence and the Conflict of Generations*. New York: W. W. Norton.

Peller, L. E. 1954. Libidinal phases, ego development, and play. *Psychoanal. Study Child* 9:178–198.

Piaget, J. 1936. *The Origins of Intelligence in Children*. New York: W. W. Norton.

Piaget, J. 1954. Intelligence and affectivity: Their relationship during child development. Palo Alto, Calif.: *Annual Reviews*. 1981.

Piaget, J. 1969. *The Psychology of the Child*. New York: Basic Books.

Pollock, G. H., 1979. Aging or aged: Development or pathology? Unpublished manuscript.

Pollock, G. 1981. Reminiscence and insight. *Psychoanal. Study Child* 36:278–287.

Rangell, L. 1963. On friendship. *J. Amer. Psychoanal. Assn.* 11:3–11.

Rangell, L. 1982. The self in psychoanalytic theory. *J. Amer. Psychoanal. Assn.* 30:863–891.

Reiser, M. 1984. *Mind, Brain, Body: Towards a Convergence of Psychoanalysis and Neurobiology*. New York: Basic Books.

Ritvo, S. 1976. Adolescent to woman. *J. Amer. Psychoanal. Assn. Supplement. Female Psychology* #5, 24:127–138.

Roiphe, H., & Galenson, E. 1981. *Infantile Origins of Sexual Identity*. New York: International Universities Press.

Ross, J. 1975. The development of paternal identity: A critical review of the literature on nurturance and generativity in boys and men. *J. Am. Psychoanal. Assoc.* 23:783–817.

Rybash, J. M., Hoyer, W., & Roodin, P. 1986. *Adult Cognition and Aging.* New York: Pergamon Press.

Sandler, J. 1960. On the concept of the superego. *Psychoanal. Study Child* 15:128–162.

Sandler, A. 1978. Psychoanalysis in later life: Problems in the psychoanalysis of an aging narcissistic patient. *J. Geriatric Psychiatry* 11(37):5–36.

Schafer, R. 1960. The loving and beloved superego in Freud's structural theory. *Psychoanal. Study Child* 15:163–190.

Seton, P. 1974. The psychotemporal adaptation of late adolescence. *J. Amer. Psychoanal. Assn.* 22:795–819.

Settlage, C. F., Curtis, J., & Lozoff, M. 1988. Conceptualizing adult development. *J. Amer. Psychoanal. Assn.* 36:347–370.

Shakespeare, W. As You Like It. In: *Shakespeare, The Complete Works* (G. B. Harrison, Ed.). New York: Harcourt, Brace, pp. 142–166.

Shane, M. 1977. A rationale of teaching analytic technique based on a developmental orientation and approach. *Int. J. Psycho-anal.* 58:95–108.

Shapiro, T., & Perry, R. 1976. Latency revisited. *Psychoanal. Study Child* 31:79–105.

Spitz, R. 1945. Hospitalism: An inquiry into the genesis of psychiatric conditions in early childhood. *Psychoanal. Study Child* 1:53–72.

Spitz, R. 1946. Anaclytic depression: An inquiry into the genesis of psychiatric conditions in early childhood. *Psychoanal. Study Child* 2:313–342.

Spitz, R. 1965. *The First Year of Life.* New York: International Universities Press.

Stern, D. N. 1974. The goal and structure of mother-infant play. *J. Amer. Acad. Child Psychiat.* 13:402–421.

Stern, D. N. 1985. *The Interpersonal World of the Infant.* New York: Basic Books.

Stevens-Long, J. 1979. *Adult Life: Developmental Processes.* Palo Alto: Mayfield.

Stevens-Long, J. 1990. Adult development: Theories past and present. In: *New Dimensions in Adult Development* (R. Nemiroff & C. Colarusso, Eds.). New York: Basic Books.

Stoller, R. J. 1968. *Sex and Gender: On the Development of Masculinity and Femininity.* New York: Science House.

Ticho, G. F. 1976. Female anatomy and young adult women. *J. Amer. Psychoanal. Assn. Supplement, Female Psychology* #5, 24:139–156.

Tyson, P. 1982. The role of the father in gender identity, urethral eroticism, and phallic narcissism. In: *Father and Child* (S. H. Cath, A. Gurwitt, & J. M. Ross, Eds.). Boston: Little, Brown.

Tyson, P., & Tyson, R. L. 1990. *Psychoanalytic Theories of Development.* New Haven: Yale University Press.

Vaillant, G. 1977. *Adaptation to Life.* Boston: Little, Brown.

Vaillant, G. 1990. Natural history of male psychological health. XII: A forty-five year study of predictors of successful aging at age 65. *Amer. J. Psychiatry* 147:31–37.

Van Gennep, A. 1908. *The Rites of Passage* (M. B. Vizedom & G. L. Caffee, Trans.). Chicago: University of Chicago Press.

Waelder, R. 1932. *The Psychoanalytic Theory of Play in Psychoanalysis: Observation, Theory, Application* (S. A. Guttman, Ed.). New York: International Universities Press, pp. 84–100.

Wallerstein, R. S. 1981. The bipolar self: Discussion of alternate perspectives. *J. Amer. Psychoanal. Assn.* 29:377–394.

Wayne, G. J. 1953. Modified psychoanalytic therapy in senescence. *Psychoanalytic Review* 40:99–116.

Wechsler, D., 1941. Intellectual changes with age. In: *Mental Health in Later Maturity*. Supplement 168, Federal Security Agency: U.S. Public Health Service.

Winestine, M. (Reporter). 1973. The experience of separation-individuation . . . through the course of life: Infancy and Childhood (Panel Report). *J. Amer. Psychoanal. Assn.* 21:135–140.

Winnicott, D. W. 1953. Transitional objects and transitional phenomena. In: *Playing and Reality*. New York: Basic Books, pp. 1–25.

Wolf, E. S. 1980. Tomorrow's self: Heinz Kohut's contribution to adolescent psychiatry. In: *Adolescent Psychiatry* (S. C. Feinstein, Ed.). Chicago: University of Chicago Press.

Wolf, E. S. 1988. Case discussion and position statement. *Psychoanal. Inq.* 8:425–446.

Wolf, K. M. 1945. Evacuation of children in wartime: A survey of the literature, with bibliography. *Psychoanal. Study Child* 1:396–404.

Yogman, M. W. 1982. Observations on the father-infant relationship. In: *Father and Child* (S. H. Cath, A. Gurwitt, & J. M. Ross, Eds.). Boston: Little, Brown.

Index